BEER BELLY BLUES

Becoming the Ultimate Male. Again

What Every Aging Man and the Women in His Life Need to Know

Cover design by Brad J. King

Illustrations by Carsten Mell

Text design and typesetting by Burnt Sky Media

Abundant Health Systems Inc.

Printed in Canada by Grafikom, Edmonton, Alberta, Canada

Grafikom is a FSC certified printing company.

FSC (Forest Stewardship Council) certification is the world's highest endorsement for environmentally and socially responsible forestry practices. By buying products with the FSC label you are supporting growth of responsible forest management worldwide.

This book is dedicated to the memory of my
father, Allan, who died of cardiovascular disease
and prostate cancer.

I wish I knew then, what I
know now.

CONTENTS

INTRODUCTION
The Invitation

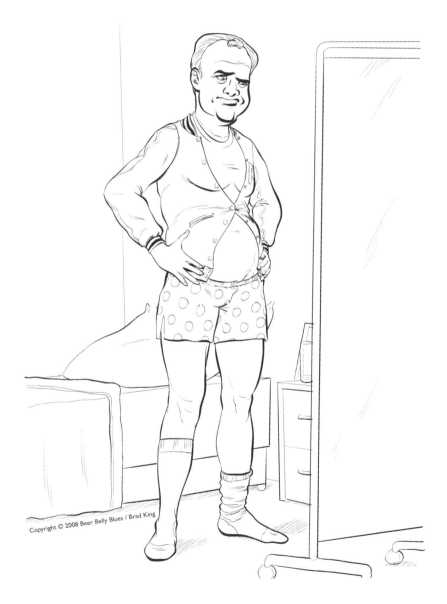

I knew this day was coming. I'd parked it in the back of my mind, which is what I do with those things over which I have no control but nonetheless dread, like property taxes and prostate exams. Lately though, every time I went out to the mailbox I'd felt a sense of impending dread, because deep inside I knew the much-prophesized moment of truth was drawing near. I realized this could be the day, and if it wasn't, tomorrow was suddenly even more likely to be. More than an envelope showing a return address from my ex-wife's attorney, even more than the once-a-year life insurance premium notice that reminds me I haven't yet changed my beneficiary, nothing, and I do mean nothing, strikes complete and utter terror into the heart of a recently-divorced man than the arrival of this one singularly inevitable and terrible thing: an invitation to your 25th high school class reunion.

Talk about a wake-up call. Or in my case, yet another wake up call.

Somehow, with that life-changing envelope clutched in my trembling hand, I managed to make it back to my front door without throwing up on the bougainvillea bushes that lined the way. Not that I'm all that into bougainvillea – I can barely spell it – it's just that since my divorce I live in a condo complex covered with the stuff.

For most of us, especially men, we really have no idea we've drifted off into the insidious slumber of middle age, or how far we've fallen from the grace of our youth. One day you're David Beckham with abs like the grill of a Bentley and an attitude to match, and twenty-five years later you wake up and you're Rush Limbaugh after a 12-day all-you-can-eat cruise. Life insurance bills I can handle, but this... no, this was a four-alarm emergency of the highest order. My self-image and my ego were being called out – they'd taken quite a beating lately, to be honest – and even if I really could run and hide from the four hundred sets of judgmental eyes that would be there, there was no hiding from the one single person who counted most: me.

Okay, make that two important people. My ex-wife would be there, too.

My first inclination, not remotely unique I'm sure, was simply to not go. To conjure up an excuse that even my ex-wife's brilliant attorney could not disprove. To move to Puerto Vallarta and take up basket weaving. But that urge quickly collided with an even stronger psychological need, this one far more noble and healthy: I wanted to go. If I could get past the paranoid notion that everyone there would be whispering, "hey, what the hell happened to him?" it would be a night to remember.

Then again, with my ex strutting her homecoming queen stuff, very possibly on the arm of another man, it just might end up being a night to jump off a bridge.

No, there was no getting out of this one. Not if I wanted to hang on to the last thin shred of self-respect I suspected still lingered within my withering, hulking shell. I was going. Now all I had to do was figure out how to transform the suddenly single old fart staring back at me in the mirror, the one with the beer belly and the receding hairline and a chin reminiscent of a turkey gullet, into some semblance of the smugly grinning jock that had been the homecoming queen's clueless but buff boyfriend. And then her husband. And then her ex-husband.

Now all I had to do was figure out how to begin the transformation.

My name is Fred, but back in school they called me The Man. Okay, they really didn't call me The Man, that was just the caption of the yearbook photo on the page announcing that I had been named Best

Athlete by a committee of my peers. You wouldn't guess it now, but back then I could throw a football sixty yards on a line and out-bench press the linemen protecting me. But fate had intervened in the form of a scalpel and a missing ACL, so I stashed my jockstrap in the attic and earned a degree in finance, took up golf, got married and have since been mired in middle management at a bank, doing what men do, raising kids and generally managing to live some semblance of the good life, give or take.

Then, doing what men do, it all went to hell in a hand basket. I had gradually let myself go, which somehow played into the sudden and complex explanation for my wife deciding that life was too short and I wasn't the ticket after all. This, of course, being what her parents had been telling her all along. So here I am in a singles city condo with a view of the industrial district, seeing my kids every other weekend, paying child support, drinking too much and exercising too little (as in, not at all), blaming everyone else for my problems, giving thanks for my wide-screen high-def plasma and a new DVR. Hey, pass the chips and salsa, life isn't so bad after all, especially with video-on-demand and the internet.

Who did I think I was kidding?

But now, with a class reunion invitation in my hand, none of that really mattered. I had twelve weeks until the Big Day, which would be held at a hotel off the freeway, dinner and dancing and a slide show that would show us all how much we'd aged. On the day the invitation arrived I made a bee-line for the closet, digging out my old letterman jacket – one of the few things I got to keep in the settlement – which hadn't seen the light of day since gas was a buck a gallon. As I put it on, or at least tried to, I realized that I was breathing hard and that my heart was racing. In fact, I was actually dizzy, since the walk from the golf cart to the tee box over the years had been about all the exercise I'd known, and even that had been a while. Of course, the jacket looked ridiculous – for a moment I thought there was a very real possibility that a few of the seams would give way before my eyes as I stood there in front of the mirror – and I was suddenly stricken with the realization that I was far, far over the proverbial hill. From a purely statistical point of view I was actually closer to death than I was the day when that jacket had fit perfectly.

It was right then when this latest threat to my ego met the abrupt dawning of my realization that not only was I out of shape and barely recognizable – thank God for reunion nametags – but I was also certainly a textbook case for an entire laundry list of impending middle age medical disasters. I'd be lucky if I even made it to reunion day.

I had twelve weeks to make all this go away.

And that was the beginning. Not just of my push to make the best of my appearance at my 25th high school reunion, but the beginning of the rest of my life, which I hoped would be longer and more pleasurable for the effort.

I knew this resurrection process would not be easy. What I didn't know was how much I really could accomplish in that time, and how high the stakes really were.

❖ ❖ ❖ ❖ ❖ ❖

Welcome to middle age. Or more accurately, to what for men is more clinically referred to as *andropause.* Women have their own term for this time of a man's life: *"Grumpy old man syndrome."* And a truer description has never been written. Andropause, or male menopause, is the hormonally-triggered decline of body, mind and spirit that manifests not only in the mirror, but in the lives of men who don't make the effort to do something about it. Unlike menopause in women, which usually begins in their mid to late-forties and hormonally decimates their child-bearing abilities, not to mention their sex drive, by the mid-fifties, men begin feeling and actually seeing the effects of mid-life hormonal change in their late thirties, some even earlier. What once was lean muscle tissue gives way to fleshy deposits of fat (to be clear, muscle does not turn into fat, any more than bone can transform itself into skin; but as muscle tissue atrophies and disappears with age, fat deposits often appear in the same location, giving the appearance of a literal trans-formation).

Lean Muscle Mass: The Key to Metabolism

This is one of the primary reasons our metabolism declines with age. Muscle is the key metabolic engine of the human body, and normal aging (or abnormal aging, depending upon how you view it) strips men of anywhere from one-third to one-half of our muscularity, which in turn causes our metabolism to slow to the pace of an inebriated snail. The extra muscle on a younger man is also the main reason why men burn up to 30 percent more calories than women — even sitting on their hairy behinds (unless they shave their butts that is, in which case they probably don't care much about muscle at all).

If most men *only* experienced a drastic decline in their ability to burn calories over a 24 hour period as they aged, that would be reason enough to get depressed. The truth, however, is worse than that, because this is really just the beginning. It all goes south from there.

Yeah, getting old sucks, and not just because our muscles, if left untended, whither away. Just how does it suck? Let us count the ways.

Singing the Beer Belly Blues

What once was a healthy, sexy head of hair gradually becomes a diminishing shadow of its former self, tinged with evidence of emerging grey. Pants and belts that once fit perfectly are suddenly snug (not to mention sorely out of style), and the statistics that define one's health – blood pressure, heart rate, cholesterol, PSA, among others – are suddenly things that must be monitored with the same devotion as the stock exchange and your kid's report card. And worst of all, the hungry sexuality that consumed your teenage years has cooled – frankly you'd rather play golf – despite the ironic fact that the woman lying next to you seems more frisky than ever, at least if you listen to how she talks to her girlfriends or gobbles up anything with Matthew McConaughey on the cover.

To state it in less than clinical terms – all of this simply and completely sucks. And while that fellow looking back at you from the mirror may be a mystery, the explanation behind the way he looks is not: as a man ages, his body loses its ability to produce the same level of testosterone that it once did. And when that happens, everything goes to hell in a hand basket, or so it seems.

It's just that simple. When testosterone goes down, things change. Bad things happen. Then we go from bad to worse. Muscles shrink, body fat percentage increases, once defined abdominal six-packs turn into a keg, losing weight becomes more difficult (if not nearly impossible), energy levels go down, hairlines recede into oblivion, erections become projects, you develop a sudden awareness of something called a prostate gland, and your wife or significant other watches the whole thing with silent, supportive horror, hoping against hope that you'll find a way to fight back. Or worse, not caring if you do because – let's get real here – she no longer is chemically attracted to who and what you've become, and those Matthew McConaughey magazines are all that she needs these days.

Like I said, it sucks.

The Good News of Hormonal Cause and Effect

For men who care about any or all of these issues – which should cover just about every guy out there with a pulse – there is astoundingly good news. Because there is a way to fight back. We can't combat the passage of time in a *chronological* sense, but we absolutely can go to war with the effects of aging in a *biological* sense, both medically and aesthetically. We really can feel better, live longer and actually look better while we're at it. Maybe not at the level of one's raging youth, but much better than all those guys on the putting green with their guts hanging over their Tommy Bahama leather-weave belts. With the right combination of lifestyle changes in the form of diet, exercise, and non-prescription supplementation, and if needed, medical intervention, hormone levels can be maintained. Which makes it far more likely that you can keep your hair, hold on to more of your lean muscle mass, and in many cases grow some new lean muscle tissue, manage your hard-on and your ego to the levels you want them to be, even approximating the way things were when you were too young to even think about such things. Because lets face it, back then you really didn't have to.

This book is about how to get this done. We'll be with Fred as he prepares for his class reunion in twelve weeks, and the inevitable showdown with his ex-wife, who indeed will be at the reunion with – and this is any man's worst nightmare – a younger, richer guy at her side, and one who looks suspiciously like – who else – Matthew McConaughey.

But don't count Fred out yet. Because the path he's about to embark upon is rich with wisdom and opportunity, and if he does the right things the right way, and makes the commitment to apply the abundant discipline required... well, his ex-wife just might have a surprise in store come reunion night.

And, so might Fred.

PART ONE

Singing the Beer Belly Blues

1

The Birth of the Beer Belly

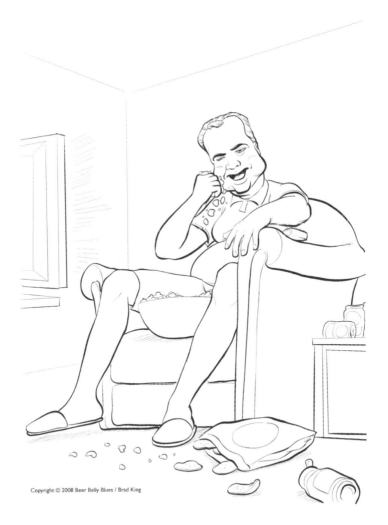

I wanted to do this right. Sure, I could have joined a weight-loss program that delivers miniscule meals to my door, maybe sign up for Hair Club for Men and get a tan, but there was more going on here than the deterioration of my body and my face, especially compared to the one shown in the high school yearbook that would be blown up and pasted on my nametag on reunion night. Beneath these significant ego issues there were other, more critical factors in play, both physiological and psychological. Given the stakes, which were nothing short of life saving, I wasn't going to leave it to those cheesy little ads in the back pages of the men's magazines I kept stashed under my bed. No, this situation called for bona fide professional help, the kind with waiting rooms, pasty white jackets and health insurance claim forms.

I know lots of guys who aren't crazy about doctors. Some are just too macho or perhaps just lazy, maybe even terrified, to darken the doorway of a physician for anything short of life-threatening symptoms. And even then, some wait too long. I'm of the mind that doctors certainly have their place, but I'm also smart enough to realize that they are more often than not the last people you want to see to get advice about how to get healthy and stay there. Having said this – and it really pissed off my wife whenever I did say this – an annual physical exam is a beautiful thing, even when the news isn't good. Actually, a yellow flag from your doctor is a gift, because at the end of the day nobody can say they didn't warn you. But the flag being waved isn't always yellow, and too seldom is it green, which is part of the issue here.

In my view at least, doctors aren't always the best option, or even the only option. We all know that when your life is on the line it's good to get a second opinion, and at the very heart of that truth is the implication and very real possibility that doctors can be wrong, or that they don't know everything, or that some are better than others. In fact, I recently read a report that was funded by a non-profit research organization called the Nutrition Institute of America, which presented compelling evidence that today's medical system frequently causes more harm than good. Now how many times have we heard that on the evening news?

The human body, for all our knowledge, is not yet an exact science. This is just as true when your life isn't on the line, if you just want to get rid of a nagging ache or two. So as I faced my twelve-week resurrection process from the precipice of social and sexual oblivion in preparation for my 25th high school reunion, not to mention a senior care center – which is how I viewed life after taking a long look at that guy in the mirror – I decided to do something a little different this time.

I decided on a team approach. Team Fred, I'd call it. I'd go back to the gym that somewhere in the depths of their computer system still showed me as a member, and I'd hire a personal trainer who looked nothing at all like Matthew McConaughey. Preferably a hot babe. I'd pay a visit to a chiropractor to work on my sciatica, which sometimes torments my calves while standing in one place. Or when I dance, which I planned to do in twelve short weeks. And I'd go see my ex-wife's naturopathic doctor – she swore by her – to talk about what I could do to address the long list of health issues that had conspired to make me look more like that infamous Nick Nolte arrest mug shot than it did the guy my wife married so long, long ago.

I had plenty of personal experience and rationale behind this choice. I'd had a bad back for years, ever since I quit playing football after I blew out my knee. My doctor did the usual round of MRIs – to the tune of four grand, which my insurance company wasn't crazy about paying; but then, they never are – before concluding I needed surgery to repair a compressed disk that was on the verge of popping. He said something about taking some tissue from my thigh and putting it in there with the disk – forgive me if I don't remember the specific protocol, but I was panicking at the time – and after about a year or so I'd feel just fine, though I'd always have to be careful about strenuous physical activity. I remember him going over all this, using the back-lit x-rays and a bunch of little diagrams for visual support, then looking straight at me and with a smug little grin, not unlike a guy I once bought a car from, asking, "So Fred, should I schedule an O.R. for you?"

Yeah, right. Sorry bub, not gonna happen. He was gonna have to score that Benz payment from some other sucker with a sore back.

I'd already noticed that doctors went mostly by the book – the one they got at medical school – every time. My blood pressure had always been around 140 over 90, which is not horrible, but not anywhere near good, either. Once I told him I preferred good to adequate, to which he responded that unless the numbers were within a certain range that warranted medication – which had risks of unpleasant side effects – there was nothing I could do. At least he mentioned the side effects. Same with my thyroid – the numbers were at the low end, but hey, better than the red zone. So no meds. Then, a few years later, the very same story came up about my cholesterol levels – not terrible, but not good. And again, no meds.

Gee, thanks doc. I knew I was definitely on my own in the preventative medicine department.

Now, I don't know about you, but I don't want to live on the fence that borders the red zone, and I don't like being told there's nothing I can do to improve the state of my health while I'm there.

(It's like being told by a financial advisor that there's nothing you can do until you declare bankruptcy. Ludicrous.) Or, if there were things I could do, they had nothing to do with medicine, so the doctor wasn't remotely interested. "If things get worse, we can take a look," was the essence of what I was told for each of these potential problem areas, and I'd been hearing it for years. "Hope you don't keel over on the golf course, call me if you do."

Not good enough. Especially for that little back spasm problem.

So I went to see my wife's naturopath. Guess what she did? She laughed. She actually laughed. She told me that the best thing I could do was lose 15 pounds and begin doing some stretching exercises, for which she gave me a video. Two months later virtually all the pain in my back was gone – I'd lost 18 pounds and my abs had mysteriously reappeared – and I hadn't experienced any back problems since. I even got an x-ray years later, and there was no evidence whatsoever of a compressed disk.

So much for booking that O.R.

Well, at least not until a few years ago. My weight had crept back up over the years and my abs had once again disappeared beneath a sea of what felt like lemon meringue under my shirt – I'd developed an affection for brie cheese and cheap white wine, and what's a ballgame without a few beers and a van full of chips? – and with it came the return of my lower back issue, which was the source of the sciatica. Not to mention the development of a gut that looked like I'd swallowed a volleyball. And oh, don't forget the hasty retreat and bleaching-out of my hairline, and a penis with a mind of its own and nowhere to go.

So now, facing 12 intense weeks of physical and emotional rehabilitation – I liked to think of it as getting ready for daily doubles in football, preparing for the season to start, in this case, the season being the rest of my life – I decided to give the naturopath another try. Team Fred would begin with her.

Heck, my regular doctor would probably just shrug and say something like, "hey Fred, you're getting old, we're all getting old, this is what happens when you get old, get used to it, play a little golf and eat fewer chips and enjoy the time you have left. And have fun at your reunion – say hi to your wife for me, she's hot."

Schmuck.

My naturopath, as it turned out, had something very different to say, indeed.

❖ ❖ ❖ ❖ ❖ ❖

A naturopathic doctor practices medicine that is complimentary to, as well as an alternative to, traditional medicine. It includes everything from chiropractic and homeopathy to herbalism, acupuncture and aromatherapy. It can even include a component of counseling that focuses on patient behavior as well as patient pathology. Naturopathic doctors take a holistic approach to their craft, applying practices and theories from different cultures and geographies, always in concert with accepted medical principles and known therapies. The hallmark of the naturopathic doctor is a preference for therapies and solutions other than synthetic drugs and invasive surgeries. Naturopathic doctors also practice prevention, which is something sorely missing in the world of allopathic (traditional) medicine. Which means Fred would not likely be told he required liposuction, an arterial splint or hair implants to get himself ready for his class reunion in twelve weeks.

What Fred did receive upon visiting his naturopathic physician was a battery of tests following an in depth discussion of his life, his goals – including the reunion – and his behaviors. His body-fat composition was taken using two methods: calipers which measure skin-fold fat contents at various points on the body, and, at a second appointment because the results of the first were a little alarming, an immersion test that uses water displacement formulas to accurately determine the percentage of fat to total body mass. His blood was also drawn to check for a variety of conditions, including traditional lipid levels (the various types of cholesterol and triglyceride readings), as well as liver enzymes, thyroid function and hormone levels.

A few days later he was back in the office to learn his results. They weren't pretty, but they weren't a death sentence, either. And best of all, they came with some very real options for therapies, behavior changes and supplementation that gave Fred a very real shot not only at buffing up for the reunion, but for beginning a path of lifelong health, increased energy, improved self-confidence and, once this was all in place, a second chance at happiness. And who know, perhaps even love.

As his new doctor went over these results with him, he realized he could have received the same data from his regular doctor. But the chances were almost nonexistent that he'd be hearing the same advice on how to respond to it – no medicines of any kind were part of this recommended regimen – or that he stood any chance whatsoever of actually changing the numbers over time. He was, after all, simply getting old.

A Focus on Flab

The thing Fred wanted to focus on, first and foremost, was his weight. Specifically, the mass of flab hanging over the front of a belt buckle that nobody had seen in a decade. Fred had a gut. Or as he and his wife had affectionately referred to it, his *beer belly*. It was matched by soft, fleshy arms and what his wife had sarcastically referred to as "back fat," those little doughy rolls on the sides that cascade down to join what is more traditionally called one's "spare tire." In Fred's case, a truck tire.

He expected a lecture on improving his diet and getting more exercise, and he did indeed hear about this as part of the solution to his concerns about weight. But he was taken by surprise by what came with this lecture – he was told that his testosterone levels were low. Very low. And this lack of testosterone was very likely one of the main factors behind Fred's spare truck tire.

Low testosterone has been linked to excess body fat – especially where the beer belly is concerned – for many years. But it wasn't until the last decade or so that studies started confirming this theory. Norwegian researchers have actually discovered that most men can determine whether they are deficient in testosterone by looking at the size of their waist. The researchers discovered that men with waist sizes greater than 40 inches had on average 30 percent lower testosterone levels than men with waist sizes that were less than 37 inches. This means that if you are presently living with a beer belly, like Fred, you are probably also experiencing low testosterone levels. Talk about a wake-up call.

Fred's testosterone levels were so low, in fact, that he was near the bottom of the normal range for men of his age. The reason the majority of aging men are not diagnosed with andropause is because blood test laboratory reference ranges are age-adjusted, reflecting the anticipated reduction in testosterone that almost all men experience. In other words, the tables accept a reduced range, in effect saying that a man should accept his decline gracefully. When it comes to optimal hormonal readings, "the normal range" doesn't exactly reflect healthy, it just fits age. And if you plan on living a long, healthy life, you need to protect your testosterone levels at all costs. In one study from the University of Washington that looked at testosterone levels in war veterans over 40, researchers found that those with the lowest levels experienced 75 percent greater death rates than the men with normal levels.

So if "normal" sucks, in Fred's words, then asking men to accept diminishing testosterone levels as they age is just plain unacceptable. Especially when they have options, which they do.

The Biochemistry of the Beer Belly

Men lose about one percent of their testosterone – the amount they produce on a regular basis – for every year they age past thirty. Which is why optimal testosterone levels should be those of a 21-30 year old, when the level was, in fact, normal and optimal. By the time they are 60 years old, men typically produce 60 percent less testosterone than they did at age 20.

The reality was that Fred, at 43, had lost about 13 percent of what had been his normal level of testosterone when he was younger. While he had heard of this depressing phenomenon before, he was surprised to learn how it affected his weight – specifically, his level of body fat and the ability, or more accurately put, inability, to gain and keep lean muscle mass. Like everyone else he'd read about athletes who took steroids to increase their level of strength, but he hadn't made the connection to percentage of body fat, which is the primary issue for men entering middle age.

The Nectar of Life

Testosterone is the nectar of life in a man's body. It is secreted by the testes (women have it too, though in much smaller quantities; healthy men produce a minimum of ten times more of it than women), and to a smaller extent, by the adrenal glands. Because men use testosterone for the maintenance of certain functions, it must be constantly replaced by the body's natural mechanism for creating it. As men get older, that natural process slows down, and thus, the levels of testosterone present in the blood gradually diminish.

The more testosterone that is present in the blood, the more prevalent and pronounced are the attributes normally associated with being a man – muscularity and strength (called anabolic function), bone strength and mass, facial hair, body hair, voice pitch, sexual drive and the performance of sexual organs. Too little testosterone and these things are compromised. Too much testosterone and, while the hairy fellow who has such a condition may be able to bench press a Buick, there comes the likelihood of other health issues.

The so-called "normal range" of testosterone for men is

a reading of 300 ng/dl (nanograms per deciliter, or the number of 1/billionth of a gram units present in 1/10th of a liter of blood) on the low end, and 1000 ng/dl on the high end. If a test scores 350 ng/dl, for example, a medical doctor is unlikely to recommend a course of action to raise the number (remember, the ranges are age-adjusted), and if he or she did, it would most likely be in the form of hormone replacement therapy via synthetic hormone shots or patches, which can have serious implications and side effects. Which means, in the absence of compensating measures, the patient is sentenced to a low testosterone life – i.e., difficulty gaining muscle mass and increasing strength, a propensity to gain body fat and difficulty in losing it, low energy, soft bones, and less than desired sexual performance. And this is just the tip of the iceberg.

Although there are much safer bio-identical hormones that can be prescribed which are identical in structure to the ones the human body produces, most doctors are unaware of these alternatives. Or if they are aware, they simply dismiss them due to a lack of substantiated research. Yeah right, let's not forget that so-called research-substantiated horse-derived hormones were used to treat menopause for years, and that thousands upon thousands of women suffered serious side-effects including heart attacks and strokes. Yet for some reason life altering side-effects are okay, as long as a pharmaceutical is backed by research.

A naturopathic doctor, however, is more likely to take a more optimistic, pro-active approach toward improving this situation, but without the use of synthetic drugs or other means that interfere with the body's natural mechanism for producing testosterone. Indeed, the solution prescribed by a body's natural ability to both produce and limit the degradation of testosterone, with no side effects other than making the patient feel like a schoolboy again.

It took Fred a while to connect this testosterone seminar to the issue of his beer belly, but he was patient and was soon rewarded with a clear understanding.

The Numbers Game

Fred's testosterone reading was 340 ng/dl, or near the low end of the range. His new doctor informed him this was normal for men in their sixties, but quite low for men in their forties. Then she explained how this related to Fred's tendency to gain and keep weight, and to store most of that excess weight around his middle. In all likelihood his regular doctor wouldn't have even broached the subject, given that Fred's declining testosterone reading fell within the age-adjusted table he was using. His naturopathic doctor, however, brought a broader view to the issue, one that gave Fred several new avenues of hope.

Without resistance exercise (lifting weights), which is required to maintain muscle mass as men and women age, muscle tissue shrinks. It's a clear-cut case of use it or lose it. The lower a man's level of testosterone, the faster that shrinkage occurs (shrinkage being a word no man wants to hear), and the slower the response when he does return to the gym and begin exercising to build the muscle back up again and regain anabolic function. In Fred's case, he'd lost a significant amount of the muscle mass that had made him a legend back in school. It was as if he'd transformed from a firm Macintosh apple into a runny apple crisp smothered in whipped cream.

Why is this important? After all, Fred wasn't going back to the locker room, and lifting weights just wasn't his thing. Who cares if he's losing a little strength? The answer to that got his attention: muscle tissue burns more than fat. A 200 pound muscular man burns off more calories – a lot more calories – in a day than a 200 pound fat guy – which may seem counter-intuitive because the fat guy seems to have to work harder to do the same amount of work. But this is nonetheless true, even if you don't move a muscle all day long. The more muscular you are, the more you can eat before it is stored as fat. Fat begets fat, and as you are now well aware, muscle burns calories to keep you from getting fat. In a very real sense, muscle is the key metabolic engine of the body. Which means, time spent in the gym is best applied to lifting weights to gain lean mass, every bit as much as doing aerobic exercise, which most people think of first when it comes to weight management. The best course of action is to do both.

Fred's percentage of body fat was 33, which put him over the line and into the obese category. His BMI (body mass index) was 31, again clearly in the high risk, obese category, just a few clicks below the morbidly obese category. He was six foot one and weighed in at 240 pounds, about 40 pounds above his playing weight back in school. Fat, sure, he'd admit that. But obese? That word had never entered his consciousness. If he had to guess, he'd say about 30 of those extra pounds were hanging around his waist. And he'd be close to correct, but in ways far more sinister than even he could imagine.

The Gradual Inflating of the Spare Tire
Many things contribute to the accumulation of body fat as men age. However, studies confirm that testosterone plays a very large role in our body's ability to either store fat or burn it.

Testosterone seems to accomplish this by first increasing the number of specific fat-releasing receptors that reside on the surface of fat cells. Secondly, testosterone inhibits a key enzyme – *lipoprotein lipase*, or LPL – that is responsible for fat storage.

Aside from this, testosterone also plays an important role in helping insulin do its job effectively. The reason this is so important is because insulin happens to be the premier fat storage hormone of the body (more on this later, in Part Two) and excess levels of it (hyperinsulinemia) are directly connected to how much fat you are able to store. The problem is that hyperinsulinemia is almost always associated with a condition known as insulin resistance, wherein the body's cells become resistant to insulin and thereby summon even more insulin into the blood. In fact, the majority of men who experience insulin resistance (which leads to Type 2 diabetes) are known to suffer from low testosterone levels. Researchers from Johns Hopkins School of Medicine in Baltimore have estimated that up to 64 percent of men who suffer from diabetes exhibit diminished levels of testosterone.

Low testosterone and excess body fat are exacerbated by diminished exercise and poor eating habits, especially the consumption of alcohol, which is one of the premiere destroyers of testosterone. Hence the term beer belly: one beer has the same calorie content as a bowl of cereal (the kind with a toy in the box), which is fine if you stick to that one beer. But if you considered eating six bowls of cereal – equal to drinking a six pack over an evening – one quickly gets a sense of context.

Alcohol and the Beer Belly

Consuming excess alcohol can stop your quest for the elusive six-pack cold (pun intended). But it does so in many more ways than just adding extra calories to your diet. In fact, only about five percent of alcohol calories ever become fat. This is due to the fact that your body will use the alcohol as energy, all the while leaving your fat right where it already resides.

It's true, calories contained in alcohol are used to fuel the body before body fat is used for that purpose. The reason for this is because of the way alcohol is metabolized. Alcohol is broken down by the liver, first into a substance called *acetaldehyde* and then into *acetate* (commonly referred to as – believe it or not – *vinegar*). Acetate is the substance that seems to prevent fat from being oxidized, or burned as energy, and acetaldehyde is a powerful testosterone inhibitor. One study appearing in the journal *Alcohol* (yes, there is such a journal) showed that one night of drinking can lower testosterone for up to 24 hours. Think about that the next time you slam down a six pack while slapping your belly with a big grin on your mug.

To support the evidence that alcohol does, in fact, contribute to the Beer Belly Blues, researchers from the University of California (Berkeley and San Francisco) embarked on a study of eight men who consumed two alcohol drinks (each containing approximately 90 calories) within a period of 30 minutes. For several hours after consuming the alcohol, the subjects ability to utilize body fat as energy declined by a whopping 73%.

If you ate the exact same amount of food every day, beginning in your thirties, you'd gradually become fat, even if that quantity of food wasn't making you fat in the early years. Why? Because your body no longer produces the testosterone required to maintain the muscle mass necessary to burn off the calories you consumed. In order to stop that slow accumulation of fat, you'd need to do several things: increase your muscle mass by engaging in a program of resistance exercise, change your diet to reduce calorie consumption and increase your protein intake, and possibly, if that didn't work, address the issue of testosterone and look for ways to increase your natural production of the hormone.

Your Muscles Don't Need to Know How Old You Are

Scientists have discovered natural ways to remain anabolic and stop the loss of muscle tissue. These include regularly performing resistance exercise and eating sufficient amounts of high-quality protein. The amazing fact is that some muscle tissue and strength loss can actually be reversed in a very short period. In 1990 a groundbreaking study appeared in the prestigious *Journal of the American Medical Association* showing muscle size and strength were greatly improved in as little as eight weeks of weight training, even in 90-year-old subjects.

Another study in the *American Journal of Clinical Nutrition* presented two groups of men aged 51 to 69 who combined resistance training only two days a week with either a meat-free diet or one containing meat, poultry, and fish. Both groups performed the same exercises. The meat eaters, who consumed approximately 16 per cent more protein, gained more muscle and strength.

Proper protein intake, especially as we age, is essential to increased protein synthesis (anabolic function). In the *Journal of Clinical Investigation*, scientists were able to increase muscle protein synthesis in elderly patients – without exercise – by giving them mixtures of amino acids, which are the building blocks of protein. The researchers concluded that increased amino acid availability can stimulate anabolic function. Therefore muscle mass can be better maintained with an increased intake of protein.

Research published in the *International Journal of Sport Nutrition* states that exercise more than doubles our need for protein. Consequently, increasing the recommended daily allowance for protein from 0.4 grams of protein per pound of body weight (0.8 grams per kilogram) to 0.8 g per lb (or 1.6 g per kg) of body weight will meet the minimum need for protein in people who exercise regularly, with weights.

Location, Location, Location

The first thing they teach you in real estate investing is that location is nine-tenths of the game. The same can be said for body fat. And you already know where the bad neighbors are in this context: your gut. Because abdominal fat is the worst kind of fat. It's literally a killer.

Body fat comes in two categories which are very different from each other, both in terms of origin and risk: *subcutaneous fat* (the fat that resides just below the skin and on top of the abdominal muscles), and the *omentum*, an actual sack-like organ deep within the abdomen that stores excess calories as fat, and can bloat to the extent that it makes a man look like he's swallowed a volleyball. With a bloated omentum, you can have a nearly rock-hard stomach that just happens to be shaped like a massive salad bowl, and is just as hard.

Omentum fat, even more than subcutaneous fat, is dangerous. It has been linked to heart disease, liver problems, cancer and diabetes, and of course, low testosterone. The presence of too much abdominal fat can obstruct the body's ability to produce insulin, which is the primary chemical governor of fat metabolism in the body. When the body fails to produce insulin – this is what happens to diabetics – it must be artificially supplemented. Failure to do so has serious health consequences, up to and including death. One of the reasons diagnosed diabetics are almost always put on strict diets is to optimize their production of natural insulin, which means they are eating with a goal of reducing stored body fat, particularly in the omentum. Remember, low testosterone is directly related to diabetes.

In Fred's case, his naturopathic doctor told him that if he didn't get his abdominal fat under control, it could kill him before he turned 60, maybe sooner. Which, he suddenly realized, was not all that far away.

Bye Bye Testosterone, Hello Estrogen

From here things go from bad to worse. Because with abdominal fat comes the production of an enzyme in the body called *aromatase*, which is responsible for converting testosterone into estrogen. Yes, *that* estrogen, the stuff of large breasts and the inclination to go power shopping. This becomes a downward spiral, because the presence of excessive estrogen inhibits the production of natural testosterone, which in turn reduces muscle mass, leads to prostate problems, a low libido, erectile dysfunction and, in some cases, cancer. In fact, it is well known that men can produce more estrogen then women by retirement age.

Estrogen conversion from testosterone is far from an aging man's only concern. Testosterone is a fat-soluble steroid hormone that is synthesized from cholesterol, which is why it (along with estrogen) needs to be transported around the bloodstream on a special carrier protein called a *sex hormone binding globulin* (SHBG). Unfortunately, once testosterone is bound to SHBG, it is unable to exert its appropriate responses upon the body (one word: erections). And the kicker is, SHBG levels increase with age, and the more fat we accumulate — especially in the belly. So if you were looking for a reason your erection isn't what it used to be, you can blame it on SHBG, among other things.

Researchers from the University of Massachusetts have discovered that on average, there is a 13% increase in SHBG per five years of aging, making it harder and harder for elderly men to maintain an optimal metabolism. A study published in the journal *Obesity Research* showed that out of 284 middle-aged men tested, low testosterone levels were discovered to be indirectly or directly related to the amount of fat the men were carrying around their midsections.

Decreased testosterone, elevated SHBG and increased estrogen levels are bad enough, but when you consider the fact that men also experience an increase in a very harmful form of estrogen with increased age and body fat levels (known as *16-alpha hydroxy estrone*), which increases the risk of prostate cancer and makes it extremely difficult to maintain a healthy metabolism, you quickly understand that most men need a little help as they age.

And, as if all this wasn't enough, Fred's doctor told him that recent studies have shown that excess abdominal fat, along with low testosterone, may be a significant contributor to the onset of Alzheimer's Disease, as well as other diminished brain functions. On the flipside, researchers have discovered that when testosterone is given to healthy men, brain function is enhanced, along with verbal memory. Because Fred's own father had fallen victim to the disease (Alzheimer's), this really got him thinking.

After going over the results of the tests, the naturopathic doctor certainly had Fred's attention. Fred had no idea how thin the ice he had been skating upon had become, and how his profile in the mirror, however disturbing, was suddenly the least of his problems. The doctor, however, reassured Fred that to a large extent most of these conditions were reversible. We can't quite turn back time and grow young again on a chronological level, but we can head in that direction biologically-speaking, where it really counts. If he adopted a completely new lifestyle and an intense commitment to fitness and a proper diet, along with some research-backed supplementation, he could lose as much as 30 pounds before the date of the class reunion rolled around.

Suddenly Fred was excited. Now if he could actually see his feet again without bending forward, he'd be ready to dance the night away. That is, if he could remember how to dance in the first place.

2

Oh, My Aching Back...and Knees...and Shoulders...

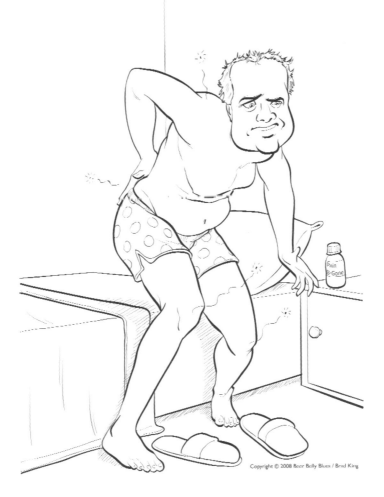

Copyright © 2008 Beer Belly Blues / Brad King

If you've every wondered what it's like to wake up from a coma, just ask me. No, I've never been in a coma, at least that I know of - my wife assured me I've been in a coma for the last two decades - but that's what my mornings are like lately. It has nothing to do with consuming too much alcohol the night before - that's more "effect" than "cause," and in my case doesn't happen all that often, at least to the extent that my hangover trumps my aching back - and it has everything to do with my past. Big time jock in school equals big time sore back in middle age, especially with a gut the size of a lawn debris bag. Or so I thought in those vague days before that class reunion invitation arrived.

How do I hurt? Let me count the ways.

My lower back felt like someone had snuck into my room in the middle of the night with a human welding device and fused the disks together into one brittle, unbendable pole. I'd wake up and swing my legs over the side of the bed, feeling around on the floor with my feet for my slippers because there was no way on God's green earth I would be able to bend over and find them with my hands. At least not if I wanted to resume an upright position any time that day. This had caused me to develop a little ritual before bed - I'd make sure my slippers were perfectly positioned for morning, just like the guys at the fire department arrange their boots and other gear for the moment when an alarm sounds off. I had an alarm of my own - it was a digital clock, and when it went off at six-thirty every morning it meant that a fire was indeed raging, in my case squarely in the base of my spine.

One word: ouch!

But getting my feet into my slippers was only the beginning of my morning ordeal. The next move was always risky, and I'd learned to keep a solid hold on the bed for a few moments to make sure it worked. I had to actually stand up. And when I did, my knees responded like a door on the Titanic – as if they had rusted shut in nearly freezing water and the hinges hadn't moved for eight decades. You could almost hear the scraping of brittle bones on tender tissue, not unlike the sound of cleaning a fish. That was the visual I had of the inside of my knees every morning, of a poor little helpless trout being eviscerated.

Other assorted aches and pains made guest appearances at less predictable intervals. My shoulders, for example, behaved as if they'd had a conference call with my knees and declared a unified front. Threading a belt through the loops of my trousers – but only after digging my waist out from the deep recesses of the folds of lard around my belly – became an exercise in sadomasochism. Reaching for something on the highest shelf of my closet – which is largely empty now for precisely this reason – required the concentration of an Olympic hurdler. I actually kept a broom in the closet for the express purpose of knocking stuff to the floor rather than have to reach for it.

All of this had conspired to create a morning ritual as embedded in my middle age DNA as the nightly slipper-positioning routine. Before even wiping the sleep from my eyes and feeling my way toward the comforting relief of plopping onto the toilet for a few minutes of blessed respite from the pain, I would gulp down four Advil tablets. Yep, industrial strength non-prescription ibuprophen. My doctor had prescribed this drug – under another name, of course – for these symptoms a few years earlier, at about twelve times the cost of the over-the-counter brand. The pharmacist told me that the prescription was merely a double strength version of the retail product, and that you could get the same effect by taking four of those pills instead of the label-recommended maximum of two.

Of course, neither my doctor nor the pharmacist ever took the time to recommend an equally or sometimes more effective natural strategy for the pain. Then again, they probably didn't know that one even existed. So I kept with the drugs even though I neglected to consult my liver on this count. Thankfully, no complaints were forthcoming... at least not yet.

This solidified two things I had long suspected – the prescription drug industry is a scam of monumental proportions, and you can't believe everything you read, even on a label.

To be honest, I had no idea if the Advil helped or not. I suspect that the pain subsided simply as a result of moving around and getting warmed up as I prepared for the day. Of course, on the so-called bad days I could always run my aching back under some hot water in the shower until I could twist from side to side (and until my hands looked like the raisins in my morning cereal). I'm usually not completely warmed up by the time I get to the stairs for the morning descent – this is why God invented handrails – but by the time I hit the door of the bank branch where I worked, I'd usually forgotten the morning's rituals in favor of a long list of awaiting headaches inside.

I had pills for those, too.

That is, except for the stomach ache. Could have been the three cups of black coffee, the extra strength vitamin pill that a good-sized horse would have trouble swallowing (which is what my doctor would have blamed it on), the lack of any real food that didn't have frosting on it, or the dissolving Advil tabs eating away the inside of my stomach lining... I had no idea.

This is why I rarely gave my football days a second thought, and hadn't for many years. Because even the slightest suggestion of throwing a football now, or God-forbid a visualization of it, even the memory of having done it once, sent shivers of agony throughout my body. Because my shoulder had enough time handling the paperwork in the bathroom, much less taking a snap from center and dropping back for a pass.

Throw a football? These days, with how my body feels, I'd rather throw up.

❖ ❖ ❖ ❖ ❖ ❖

While Fred feels singularly unique in his situation because of his history as an athlete, the fact is he's not as alone in this painful situation as he'd like to believe. In fact, many men entering middle age begin to feel the aches and pains of getting older, usually in their knees, back and often in their shoulders. It's called *osteoarthritis*, or more commonly known as realizing how fragile you are, and it's as common as gray hair in men experiencing the ravages of andropause (male menopause), which can begin as early as the late thirties.

Oh My Aching Back

The cause of osteoarthritis truly is nothing other than the passage of time. Over the years the body simply wears out, the connective tissue and especially the cartilage that comprises the complex engineering of our joints wears down, and too often wears out. An entire cottage industry in the medical profession does nothing other than replace hips, knees and shoulders, and does it with surprising effectiveness, as the body hardly tells the difference between bone, plastic and gleaming chrome, or at least this is what we are led to believe. For instance, many knee replacements are made with cobalt chrome, despite the fact that it is known to cause allergic reactions in some individuals, and otherwise is not exactly the most compatible substance with the human body. This is why newer materials like zirconium – one of the most bio-compatible elements known to man – are now starting to be used more and more.

In addition to wear and tear, though, a man's joints are challenged and compromised by the effects of inflammation. Inflammation is the common consequence of any of the over 100 varieties of arthritis (osteoarthritis, while the most common, is only one of them), but can also result from infection, injury, allergies and other causes. Although common belief holds that there is little we can do to reverse the effects of wear and the osteoarthritis it causes, short of mitigating the pain itself, research shows that cartilage destroying inflammation and rebuilding of the cartilage itself can indeed be addressed, and without prescription medicines and their side effects.

Swallow at Your Own Risk

The most common and easily accessible remedies for painful joints and an aching back are over-the-counter painkillers, especially those with anti-inflammatory properties. These are called NSAIDs – non-steroidal anti-inflammatory drugs – the most famous of which, at least for this application, is Advil and Aleve.

Here's the down and dirty science behind it all: the body produces chemicals (called prostaglandins, produced by certain enzymes stimulated by specific conditions) that serve to protect the stomach lining from acid while supporting the formation of blood clotting platelets. But there's a price for that protection. Inflammatory enzymes with crazy names like *cox* and *lox* can cause some prostaglandins to promote pain and inflammation in the joints, and cause fever. NSAIDs mostly block the production of prostaglandins, thus reducing pain and fever. But, since NSAIDs also block the so-called "good" prostaglandins that protect the stomach lining, the pills actually create a higher probability of ulcers and the pain that comes with it. A stomach ache from taking Advil, for example, may not yet be an ulcer, but it does directly relate to acids irritating the lining of the stomach

Beyond the gastrointestinal damage, many NSAIDs also inhibit the production of a major component of connective tissue called a glycosaminoglycan (GAG). GAGs are made up of long chains of proteins and sugars that work to lubricate your joints and protect them from daily wear and tear. Researchers from the Kennedy Institute of Rheumatology in London studied regular users of NSAIDs and observed a general reduction in the metabolic activity of the cells responsible for manufacturing GAGs. This means that the very medications that millions of arthritis sufferers have relied upon day in and day out to help reduce their suffering have actually been implicated in the destruction of cartilage, which leads to a further progression of the arthritic disorder for which they are initially taken. Now *there's* some serious irony.

NSAIDs aren't inherently evil, as they are a viable means of dealing with the pain of headaches, arthritis, injuries and menstrual cramping. The problem comes, especially for men, when they are used regularly to alleviate the pain of deteriorating joints caused by the natural process of aging, with the side-effect of wreaking havoc on the lining of the stomach and the eventual further destruction of the very cartilage you are trying to protect. Aside from this, they can also cause diarrhea, vomiting, loss of appetite, constipation, skin problems, headaches, heart attacks, dizziness and sleep disorders. Asthma suffers have a particularly higher risk of side effects. While many believe that ibuprophen (Advil, Aleve and Motrin) are the most famous NSAIDs, this can be disputed, since simple *aspirin* is also at the top of the list of this classification of drugs. It's easy to get, cheap, and where joint pain is concerned, it can help. But with those potential side effects, it may not be the optimal solution.

Elbows and Knee Joints and Hips, Oh My!

By now you may be wondering if testosterone or lack thereof is associated in any way with the deterioration of our joints. The answer is, in some cases, *yes*. Studies have long shown an association with low testosterone levels and rheumatoid arthritis (RA). Unlike wear-and-tear osteoarthritis, RA is believed to be an autoimmune disease that causes the body's immune system to produce antibodies against human tissue — in this case, your cartilage. It has long been known that people who suffer from RA have very low testosterone levels. According to a British study appearing in the journal, *Annals of Rheumatic Disease*, testosterone replacement is able to improve arthritic symptoms in those with RA. It turns out that the same inflammatory chemicals seen elevated in those experiencing RA, are in fact the same ones seen in men who have low testosterone levels.

Essential Fats—A Natural Alternative to NSAIDs

Consciously or not, if you, like Fred, are presently suffering from the pain and inflammation of osteoarthritis, and the damage is accumulating; it's time to give your body the supplies it needs to fight the on-going damage. And no, this doesn't include harmful cartilage-destroying drugs.

Scientists in the 1970s were baffled to discover that the inhabitants of the Arctic ate a traditional diet made up primarily of fat in the form of seal blubber, but they did not seem to suffer from any of the diseases associated with a high-fat diet elsewhere in the world. Scientific curiosity about this phenomenon, which was called the "Greenland Paradox," led to a much more sophisticated analysis of dietary fat, and soon we were hearing about "good" fats and "bad" fats. Who knew? The discovery of the "good fats" Omega-3, Omega-6, and Omega-9 changed the way we thought about eating forever (again).

When we speak of the "good" fats, what we are in fact speaking of is the Omega-3 family of essential fatty acids found primarily in, flax seeds and oil, hemp seeds and oil, almonds, walnuts, fish, algae and krill oil. Civilizations from the days on the Tigris River until now have benefited from these powerful anti-inflammatory fats. Today, the most popular form of Omega-3s are found in fish oil, however the fish that is used to make the majority of fish oil products is a far cry from the fish consumed many, many years ago. Today's fish contain traces of contaminants like mercury, PCBs and dioxins and even though modern processing methods claim to remove the majority of these toxins, one has to still wonder about the true quality of most fish oil products. This is where krill oil comes in.

Krill oil, which comes from small shrimp-like crustaceans living in the oceans off the West coast of Vancouver Island, Russia, and Japan, contain a special form of the Omega-3 fatty acids EPA and DHA (found in fish oil). But unlike other marine oils where the fatty acids are in a triglyceride form, Krill oil contains fatty acids in the form of phospholipids, which, according to studies, allows the EPA and DHA fatty acids to be better absorbed into your cells than fish oils. Krill also contains a unique but powerful antioxidant and immune-supporting carotenoid not found in fish oils, called *astaxanthin*. Aside from harboring incredible antioxidant potential (when measured by the well-accepted ORAC or Oxygen Radical Absorbance Capacity measurement), Krill was found to be 300 times more effective at quenching harmful free radicals than either vitamin A or vitamin E, 48 times more effective than fish oil, and 34 times more effective than Coenzyme Q10. Krill oil's bioavailable EPA and DHA fatty acids help to extinguish excess inflammation by competing with pro-inflammatory fats, and in the process blocking the activity of the inflammation producing COX-2 enzyme. By blocking excess inflammation, joints are able to repair themselves more effectively and help you become more mobile.

The above natural therapy is what Fred's naturopath recommended to help him deal with his back and joint pain, but without risk to his stomach lining or the possibility of further damage to his ailing joints. She may not be able to send Fred back to the stadium to throw a football like he used to, but she can send him to the reunion with knees and a back that can handle all the dancing he wants... and maybe more.

3

The Dreaded Rubber Glove

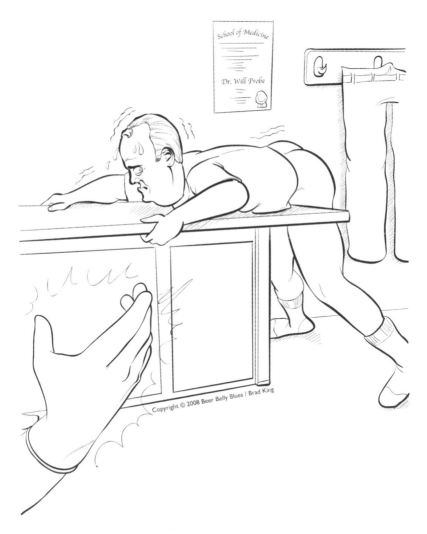

School of Medicine

Dr. Will Probe

Copyright © 2008 Beer Belly Blues / Brad King

There is a certain word out there that scares the hell out of me. And I'm pretty sure it strikes terror into the heart of any man with half a brain, or any man who, like me, has to get up numerous times in the middle of the night to pee. It's not a word you hear bandied about in casual conversation – if it is, try another bar – nor is it a word any man under the age of 40, unless he's been to medical school, gives much thought to. The word has implications and dark potential that make it easy to avoid. But you can't avoid it for long. Because after 40, there's a doctor somewhere out there slipping on a rubber glove to remind you, and no man can forget about that.

Of course I'm talking about the dreaded prostate gland, that walnut size chunk of life-altering tissue buried somewhere deep in your lower body cavity and accessible only in one of two ways: with a scalpel or that insidious, menacing rubber glove.

I realize that the prostate gland, in and of itself, is not a terrible thing. I'm not exactly sure why or how, but it does something that facilitates sexual activity, and that alone makes it one of the good guys. But I also know it has a tendency to go on the fritz, and that's the scary part. Because when that happens – everything from multiple visits to the john in the night, to serious disease, impotence and even death can occur – no other organ in the body is more important. When that happens, that's all a man can think about.

There are two things I try not to dwell too much on these days - my bowel movements and my prostate. But when I'm standing there in my bathroom in the quiet of the night, butt-naked in the dark, leaning forward with one hand on the wall and the other steering the reluctant output of my urinary plumbing toward its intended porcelain destination – not always easy to hit at three in the morning – it's a difficult thought to avoid. The bad news is that there's a history of prostate cancer in my family, which means every nocturnal call of nature wears a black robe in my mind.

Now, I know some guys have prostate issues that have nothing at all to do with cancer, theirs might just be swollen to the size of a casaba melon, but in either case it's nothing to take lightly. So I don't. When I visited my naturopath I brought a list of things I wanted to discuss in with me. And at the top of it was that singular dreaded word.

Hey, it isn't just about getting up to pee once too often, or even about the dreaded "C" word. Fact is, I don't plan on staying single forever – especially after the next 12 weeks of transformation – and with even the possibility of the slightest connection between my prostate and my ability to conjure up a world class woody, I wanted to get this on the agenda right up front.

I did rethink all this for a moment when my new doctor – a woman, and an attractive one at that, which made things worse – withdrew a rubber glove and some lubricant from the drawer. This was a whole new world of confusion. It was bad enough when my regular doctor, whose hands looked like those of a longshoreman, did the same thing... but this... I don't know. Life is complicated sometimes, and this moment proves it.

Thank God for short fingernails. At least in her case.

❖❖❖❖❖❖

Fred is right, certainly about those short fingernails, and at least about one other thing: nothing strikes fear into the heart of middle aged men quite like a conversation about his prostate gland with a doctor. And with good reason. Prostate cancer is the number two cancer killer of men in the civilized world after colon cancer, and third overall killer (after heart disease and colon cancer).

That's the bad news. The good news is that it's easy to detect and, after detection, is one of the slowest growing of all the cancers. Which means if caught early it can be treated. The survival rate for men diagnosed with prostate cancer within five years of initial onset is very high, nearing 100 percent. But beyond five years, if the cancer has spread to other organs, the survival rate drops to 38 percent. According to recent cancer statistics, prostate cancer is now being diagnosed in men at the same rate as breast cancer in women. For any man paying attention – and all men should – this is a wake up call of the first order.

Age Discrimination

The reason prostate cancer targets middle aged men has everything to do with the hormonal changes that occur in middle age, specifically, an increasing amount of estrogen in conjunction with a declining production of testosterone. In that case, the body uses a by-product of testosterone called *dihydrotestosterone* (DHT), which is widely implicated in the onset of prostate disease.

The prostate gland plays a role in the need to urinate frequently because it resides at the exit of the bladder, actually surrounding the urethra – the tube that carries urine and sperm from the body – like a donut. When the prostate swells, it partially cuts off the urinary tract leading to the penis, which means the bladder doesn't completely empty, which in turn creates the on-going need to urinate and/or a constant feeling that the bladder is never empty. If prostate swelling can be reduced, then urinary problems are relieved.

The prostate gland is also integral to healthy sexual function, as it contributes to the fluid that comprises a man's ejaculate fluid, including a chemical that causes the female genital tract to contract, thus helping to transport sperm toward the uterus through the Fallopian tubes. This is one of the reasons that many men who experience prostate swelling also experience sexual problems such as erectile dysfunction (which we'll cover in more detail later).

Another fluid produced by the prostate is called *prostate specific antigen*, more commonly known as PSA, which also plays a role in this sperm-to-uterus process. Because a small amount of PSA is present in the bloodstream, it can be measured with a blood test.

The PSA Test

When the prostate swells, more PSA is produced by virtue of the presence of a larger surface of the organ. Prostate disorders can also cause leakage of PSA into the blood-stream, which is why a PSA test may or may not be an indicator of the presence of disease. Unfortunately the PSA test has one of the highest error rates of any medical test today, often misdiagnosing patients. For every six biopsies ordered because of a PSA reading, only one cancer is discovered. According to a leading urology journal, most men who score high on the PSA test turn out *not* to have cancer at all, just an elevated level of PSA.

Despite problems with the test, urologists believe hat when a PSA score returns very high, the chances of the presence of cancer go up, since cancer causes the most PSA to be present in the blood as compared to a simple non-disease prostate enlargement. So what is normal? An index score of 1.0 is considered normal, while any reading over 4.0 is considered cause for concern. Just as concerning is the upward movement of the score over a short period of time, even if that score remains below 4.0. If your score doubles from 1.0 to 2.0 within a year, start paying attention, even though you are well below the 4.0 threshold.

The reason behind the intrusive rubber glove exam – the doctor is feeling the prostate itself for firmness, which in conjunction with the PSA test is a better indicator of potential disease – is that neither it nor the PSA test is definitive. Only a biopsy – surgical extraction of tissue from the prostate for lab testing – can return a definitive diagnosis, however a second and even third opinion is always a smart choice before allowing a piece of you to be removed and examined, no matter how small that piece may be.

Most men experience some prostate enlargement as they get older. Hence, more frequent trips to the bathroom, especially at night. About one in ten men undergo surgery to remedy a prostate condition, the other nine relying on powerful medications with numerous side-effects. As you will see later in this book, there are many natural, side effect-free options to effectively shrink a swollen prostate gland, some just as effective as side effect-prone medications.

Prostate Cancer and the Odds

About one in six men are diagnosed with prostate cancer. Older men have a higher frequency of prostate cancer than middle aged men – it has been said that if a man lives long enough, he has a 98 percent chance of the onset of prostate cancer. In most cases men don't live long enough for prostate cancer to claim their lives. This is due to the fact that the disease is among the slowest growing of all the cancers, and thankfully, at least the majority of the time, never makes its way out of the prostate to metastasize to the surrounding tissues.

Fred's fears of impotency because of prostate problems become valid only when cancer enters the conversation. The reason is that surgery removes the muscular mechanism necessary for ejaculation, and potentially damages the nerves that affect the penis, since they are in close proximity. This is why one should exhaust all other options before submitting to prostate surgery, or for that matter, any other invasive treatment. Many physicians believe the prostate grows in the presence of an increased level of testosterone; however research indicates that this is not necessarily the case.

Testosterone versus DHT

It is extremely important not to confuse testosterone with the very powerful dihydrotestosterone (DHT) that is implicated in prostate growth and cancer, as countless studies show that the prostate gland receptors have no choice but to bind to DHT when serum testosterone levels are low. It is actually high levels of DHT and the primary estrogen, *estradiol*, as well as its powerful metabolite *16-alpha-hydroxyestrone*, which contributes greatly to prostate disease and cancer. In fact, the considerable decline in testosterone men experience with age almost exactly parallels the increase in estrogens and prostate disease (BPH, prostatitis and cancer). You don't see too many twenty year old men at the peak of their testosterone production complaining about BPH or being diagnosed with prostate cancer, and the correlation is inescapable.

Unfortunately treatment for cancer often includes the deprivation of testosterone – both surgically through the removal of testosterone-producing glands, and through pharmaceutical means – called *anti-androgen therapy*, which is often associated with muscle and strength loss, depression, nausea, breast enlargement (gynecomastia), diarrhea, anemia, diminished libido, erection problems, liver problems and osteoporosis. In other words, all the symptoms of growing old, feeble and becoming only a faint shadow of one's former self. Hey, aren't these the same symptoms associated with andropause? You bet they are. Once again, before submitting to this kind of treatment, do yourself a favor and get a few more professional opinions.

The Second Opinion

In a study appearing in the prestigious *Journal of the American Medical Association*, researchers from Harvard Medical School evaluated seventy-seven men (average age of 64) with low total testosterone or free testosterone levels, with PSA levels of 4.0 ng/mL or less. The study showed that those with the highest testosterone levels fared the best and were the longest lived. Also, a high prevalence of biopsy-detectable prostate cancer was identified in men with low total or free testosterone levels. Another Harvard Medical School study looked at the association of free and total testosterone in regards to prostate cancer in 117 patients and found that low, *not* high, serum free testosterone may be a marker for more aggressive disease. And finally (although there are many, many more studies that show how important testosterone is to a healthy prostate) researchers from St. Bartholomew's and The Royal London Hospital School of Medicine reviewed 34 published studies and concluded there has so far been no conclusive evidence that levels of circulating testosterone in individuals developing prostate cancer are higher than in controls. The researchers stated, "Firstly, prostate cancers arising in men with low serum testosterone levels are more malignant and frequently non-responsive to hormones."

This is definitely something for men to think about, even when they'd rather be thinking about other things, perhaps even their upcoming class reunion.

4

Addicted to Love... But Now I'm Sober

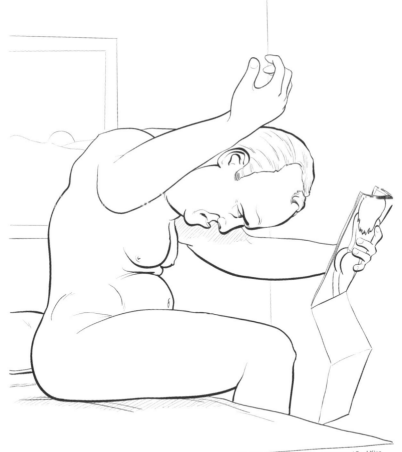

Nature can certainly be a cruel mistress sometimes. Take women, for example (many of whom can also be a cruel mistress, but that's another story). For the first 40 years of their lives their interest in sex is as much mental and social – and in some cases economic – as it is based on some deep dark physical drive, like it is in men. At least that's what I'd been told – by my wife, mostly – it's what I've read, and it's certainly been my experience. And don't forget the procreation aspect of the subject, either. Maybe that's why women kick into a higher sexual gear as they near menopause, its nature telling them that the clock is ticking.

It isn't that women don't like sex in their 20s and 30s. They do. It's just that they don't like it as much – my opinion – or for the same reasons, that men like it. Or better put, need it. That's the operative word here – need. In the first half of their adult lives men need sex, women don't, though they may choose to have it and enjoy it when they do. The point is, it's their choice.

Men, on the other hand, depart their pre-pubescent years on fire with raging sexual hunger, a walking hard-on on wheels, their minds never far from the gutter, their intentions rarely pure, their carnal needs never satisfied. It's been said that men think of sex at a rate of about once every twenty-six seconds, but I'm sure this averages in sleep time, since this seems a little thin to me. Then, just as the woman in their lives is getting into the swing of things as she looks 40 squarely in the eye, men begin to slow down on this particular issue.

For men, this is a little like winning the lottery at the age of 89.

It's all hormones, of course, which is why I blame nature for this unfortunate timing. Most couples are lucky to get about two years of hormonal compatibility at the peak of their sexual powers, or at least a mutual interest in multiple orgasms, and hopefully they can bank enough earth-shaking sexual experiences to last a lifetime of remembering the good old days. Quickly, though, it becomes apparent that the man's days of multiple orgasms and sense of adventure are dwindling – suddenly a schedule is important, as is a flat-screen in the bedroom – and soon the entire sexual context of the relationship is reversed, made all the more complicated by the fact that only one out every ten thousand couples actually sits down and talks about it (my statistic, based on research involving a control group consisting of one couple: my wife and I).

Unfortunately my wife and I missed that particular window of time. She didn't get horny until she moved out.

In the months before my divorce, especially after my wife flew the coup with the announcement that she needed more physical affection than I seemed interested in, or capable of, providing, I spent a lot of time pondering this cruel twist in the natural order of things. And I had to admit, my mental sexual meter had gone from once every 26 seconds to about once every 26 days, though I blamed the fact that my wife and I hadn't seen each other naked for the two years prior to our separation. This, of course, led me to the conclusion that it was all my fault, just as she claimed, though as I said, I much prefer to blame Mother Nature instead.

Maybe Mother Nature could pay the alimony, too.

I could play the victim role here and say that if my wife wanted sex from me she should have said something, or God-forbid, done something, but that wasn't the real issue. No, she was much too astute and sensitive to let something as obvious as communications get in the way of her next orgasm (which, I found out later, had been facilitated by a battery operated device obtained at a women's-only "gift party"). My wife knew my sexual well was going dry, and that it wasn't because of anything she'd done (which, in retrospect, was why she didn't think to even try anything close to seduction). I was just getting old, my hormones had dried up – her words, after the fact – and, as she said when she walked out the door, life is just too short to settle.

And now, facing 12 weeks of reinvention in preparation for my class reunion, I had to agree with her.

I couldn't wait to hear what my naturopath had to say about this one.

❖ ❖ ❖ ❖ ❖ ❖

It didn't take Fred long to become aware there was a theme running rampant throughout the list of issues that were troubling him about his impending middle age. All of them especially his waning libido and the unpredictable performance of his sexual plumbing – are connected to the reality that his testosterone production was slowly, but surely, winding down.

How Low Can You Go?

Low libido (along with other sexual problems, including erectile dysfunction and premature ejaculation), is unfortunately often experienced in silence. A 2002 article appearing in the *Wall Street Journal* indicated that 80 percent of men never seek treatment for their condition.

Any discussion about libido (sexual desire), as well as performance (erections and their sustainability), cannot be simplified to a singular focus on testosterone. Many couples of all ages engage in healthy, satisfying sexual relations even though they are at the low end of the normal hormone range for their age. The sexual dynamic within a couple is as much energized by the state of the relationship and the effort they put into it. Sex between older couples is often the natural outcome of a choice they've made to remain intimate and loving, even romantic and perhaps playful (and in a few rare cases, downright kinky), and to please each other in the process.

That said, though, it certainly does help if there's enough testosterone in the man's system to keep him interested in the game, and able to swing the bat once he's in the lineup.

Hard Facts

The relationship between testosterone and a healthy erection has been scientifically documented. Testosterone is a well known promoter of nitric oxide (NO), which is required for optimal blood flow (restricted blood flow is one of the reasons behind erectile dysfunction). Testosterone is responsible for stimulating nitric oxide within the expandable erectile tissues, called the *corpora cavernosa*. Research presented in the *Journal of Sexual Medicine* indicates that aside from its powerful arousal qualities, testosterone can also improve erectile function by restoring the blood-trapping capacity of blood vessels within the penis. The same journal presented a study showing that testosterone therapy was even more effective when combined with the erectile dysfunction drug, sildenafil citrate (Viagra®).

While many experts believe that low testosterone is

responsible for almost all erectile dysfunction, that fact has not yet been conclusively proven in an objective scientific laboratory. In fact, other conditions, such as heart disease (especially the narrowing of blood vessels), can also play a direct – and sometimes an indirect – role in erectile dysfunction. The interesting thing (as you will see in a later chapter) is that even cardiovascular health has a connection to healthy testosterone levels. There is also evidence that those who suffer from prostate disease also have a higher propensity to suffer from erectile dysfunction. It is no mere coincidence that prostate disease and erectile dysfunction go hand in hand. The prostate is an integral player in a man's sexuality, and proper ejaculation is dependent upon the health of this gland. In fact, the prostate is so important that half of all men who suffer from prostate disease also suffer from erectile dysfunction.

Since low levels of testosterone have a substantial effect on the quality and sustainability of erections, it is important that the issue be viewed holistically.

It is also well known that testosterone levels in men have a direct relationship with muscular size, strength and responsiveness, which can and probably does impact a man's sexual response. A healthy muscular and energized man is more likely to be sexually interested and involved than a man who isn't, so in that sense testosterone has a direct bearing on a man's quality of life.

Aside from its role in helping to achieve and maintain an erection strong enough for intercourse, testosterone also plays a role in male libido. Many scientific studies bear this out. Surveys of men on hormone replacement therapy are quick to verify that they do, indeed, sense a markedly heightened interest in all things sexual, which is not always good news for their post-menopausal partners. And since the reverse has been established scientifically – the absence of testosterone definitely negates the possibility of a chemically-inspired sexual desire, if not an emotional one – then the conclusion is clear if not exactly evident in an accredited white paper: testosterone and sex are inextricably linked.

Testosterone: Man Fuel

Even though testosterone is produced primarily in a man's testes, it has a direct relationship to the human brain. Other body functions that rely on the presence of testosterone, include the development of facial and body hair, muscular development and strength, and the body's ability to process chemicals (such as cholesterol and adrenalin) that are completely managed by the brain. And while production does indeed take place in the testes, it does so only upon a signal from the brain.

Since the sexual urge and the chemicals that give it wings almost always begins in the brain – sight, sound, touch, the perception of specific other stimuli – then it is easily concluded that woman are correct after all, sex *begins* in the brain, and depends on the perceptions that occur there to be successful. This said, it's hard to deny the role of testosterone in all aspects of the sexual equation.

Fred can rest easy wondering if his new naturopathic doctor understands all this, not to mention what's at stake. Come reunion night, he'll be a new man, in more ways than one.

5

Looking for Hair in All the Wrong Places

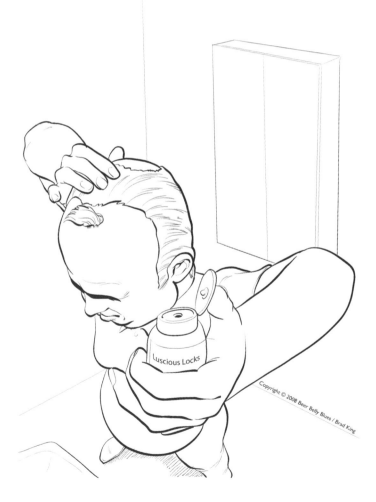

I gotta say, Doctor McDreamy (the television character with the stethoscope and the matinee idol hair) has nothing on me, at least when I was younger. Upon commenting to my soon-to-be ex-wife that I thought my hair was every bit as cool as that guy's (this being one of many pathetically weak moments just prior to our separation; I was hoping she'd throw me a bone), she said perhaps this was true, she hadn't really paid much attention lately – that punch landed – and even so, too bad it wasn't also true for my face, body and salary, as well. She didn't smile when she said it. Five minutes later she added wardrobe and sense of humor to the list. Such are the winds of impending marital discord – instead of a bone she'd heaved a tire iron – and such is the lot of many men in middle age, at least where their hair is concerned.

There's nothing at all I can think of to say about the loss of one's hair that is remotely positive. You can cover your sagging gut with a parka, you can trim the hair growing out of your ears with a battery-driven appliance that looks like a sex toy, but who the hell wants to go around wearing a baseball hat all the time? Nobody I know, or at least nobody I know who's over the age of twenty, thinks they look good in a cap with the logo of a heavy equipment manufacturer on it. I wore one to church last Easter and the minister actually mentioned it in the sermon. Being bald as a newborn pig's ass may work for the occasional hockey star or that guy who sucked a lollipop on television in the 70s, but in my view bald isn't beautiful, it's embarrassing. Oh I know, I shouldn't have my ego so darn tied up in how I look, but I ask you: what the hell should I have it tied up in? My 1998 Toyota? My wife's not stupid, she knew precisely where to toss that tire iron.

Actually, going completely bald wouldn't be as bad as what I'm dealing with these days. My hair looks like someone ran out of gas while they were mowing a putting green. There's a perfectly round patch of smooth skin on the back of my skull, as if my barber had used the bottom of a peanut butter jar to draw a perfect circle, into which was poured industrial strength chemicals. Then there's the front, where an isolated island of hair the size of a poker chip resides, completely surrounded by gleaming white skin, as if it had broken off from the mass of fuzz that appears to be receding into the horizon and is falling forward from the force of gravity, as if to meet my eyebrows, which lately are as thick as a year-old toothbrush. And then to top it off (excuse the pun), the whole receding mess is the color of the water in a bucket just after you've finished washing your car after a road rally in the foothills.

Now, you might be thinking that if this bothered me so much, why not do something about it? Good question. I was hoping my new naturopathic miracle worker would have an answer for that one, and that it had more going for it than the brand names with the bad advertising, namely Rogaine and Propecia.

❖ ❖ ❖ ❖ ❖ ❖

Fred is certainly not alone in wondering where his hair has gone, and why. Roughly one out of two men begin losing their hair at some point in their life, most in the form of what is called male pattern baldness, which is your basic receding hairline accompanied by thinning on the crown, and up to 20 million men are considered downright bald.

Just Say Bald

The more formal name for male pattern baldness is *Alopecia Areata* (which, not so coincidentally, rhymes with Propecia, a popular product created to combat it). Alopecia Areata is actually an autoimmune condition wherein the body gets it wrong – it reacts to hair follicles as if they are unwanted foreign bodies, thus preventing their growth on the affected part of the body. When Alopecia Areata is active, the hair falls out to reveal a smooth patch of skin. The good news is that Alopecia Areata can be treated, and to a great extent, even prevented.

Hair loss has also been linked to diet, but then again, what hasn't? Crash diets – otherwise referred to as *fad diets* – in particular can lead to protein deficiencies, which in turn can cause hair loss, which once again makes a lot of sense when you consider that hair, like skin, nails, and nearly everything else in your body, is mostly made of protein. Some common medications for conditions such as depression, arthritis and heart disease (including elevated blood pressure) can have the side effect of hair loss. In addition, illness and infection – not to mention simply not eating right (as in not enough protein) – can cause a depletion of protein in the body, which can result in thinning hair, as well.

Most of these conditions can be easily reversed – go off that crazy diet, start chugging down some protein drinks (see the Appendix II for some of the best), change your prescription or just get well – all without the need to drop significant money on over-the-counter products that promise to make you look like an extra from *Grey's Anatomy*.

The Real Cause of Hair Loss

In the conversation about hair loss, though, most of these issues are just white noise. Because the real culprit is the presence of too much DHT – a condition called androgenetic alopecia – and/or the inability of the body to process it. DHT results when an enzyme (5 alpha reductase) begins to convert regular testosterone into dihydrotestosterone (DHT) – if this sounds familiar, it should, because it's the same culprit in the prostate cancer discussion – to which the body has numerous adverse reactions. In fact, the aging process itself can be largely attributed to too much DHT and estrogen, and the extent to which this conversion can be slowed or prevented is the extent to which anti-aging regimens (or more commonly known as *longevity* regimens) become successful. If a man's genetic code results in a higher than normal amount of DHT in his system, or if it makes his hair follicles susceptible to the effects of DHT, the bald father is destined to beget a bald son.

It doesn't take a rocket scientist, or a naturopathic physician for that matter, to see the solution: go to war on DHT. Block it, inhibit it, send it to the showers. Non-prescription DHT blockers are available at your local health food store, not to mention all over the internet, but care must be taken when one begins to tinker with the body's natural endocrine (hormone) systems. In other words, make sure you know what you are buying. It is also interesting to note that some men respond positively to well-formulated prostate products, which contain various combinations of nutrients that help lower or block DHT production. Later in this book, we'll review some of these incredible nutrients, and in Appendix II you'll find one of the best prostate-specific formulas available today.

Thankfully Fred's naturopath has recommended one of these safe and effective remedies to help him hold onto whatever hair he has left. Who knows, Fred may even be lucky enough to experience some new hair growth before the reunion.

6

Dude Look Like a Lady

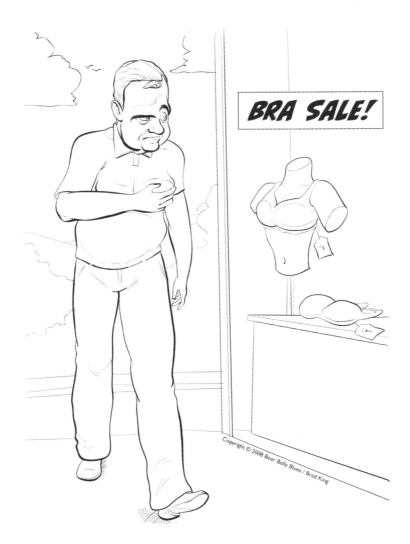

I used to love that song. You know, the one by the rock group whose members are older than dirt and whose lead singer looks like a cross between Mick Jagger and Angelina Jolie. Like most guys, I never paid much attention to the lyrics – until recently I thought "Louie Louie" was a tune about a salad – I just liked the groove, and hey, it was Aerosmith, so how uncool would digging the lyrics be, right? Until one night coming home in the car as it was playing, my wife started laughing hysterically as she watched me silently mouth the words, and when I asked why, she eagerly explained the source of her amusement. It was the irony of me liking that particular song. When I pressed for more information – rarely a good idea in the tense days prior to a divorce – she announced that my breasts were now actually larger and fuller than hers, and she was a healthy 34C who looked just fine in a bikini. This was a little bit like me telling her the hair on her upper lip was beginning to resemble a moustache, which wasn't the case, though that was precisely my response. You can imagine where the conversation went from there.

Dude look like a lady, my ass. Not this dude.

Of course, the second we got home I found a discreet mirror and took off my shirt. There they were, two ripe little melons where my pecs used to be, each with a tidy little fold of flesh – okay, it was fat – hanging down with just enough bulk to form a crease under each. Is it still a boob if it's on a man? Whatever you want to call them. Even the nipples had distended under the pressure from beneath, giving it a sort of feminine profile that frankly scared the hell out of me. Other than an affection for brie cheese, I'd had no sudden urges to watch "The View" or arrange a centerpiece for the dining room table, so this man-boob thing was completely, to use a most masculine metaphor, out of left field.

A quick trip to the computer and a search under the terms

"man boobs" and "bitch tits" (distasteful, I agree, but I'd been in enough weight rooms to know that's what the sweaty guys who hang out there call them) yielded the cold-blooded medical truth about my chest – I had something called "gynecomastica," which sounds like a cross between a math class and an island off the Grecian coast. My first impulse had been to write my fleshy lobes off to the fact that I was overweight, and certainly that was contributing to the situation. But I couldn't deny what I would never admit, not to my wife or my divorce lawyer – the tissues around my breast had been swelling like a puffer fish for some time now, and even when I'd dropped ten pounds last year on a whim, my breasts still looked disproportionately feminine.

No, this was more than too many corn dogs and a lack of proper exercise. This was positively hormonal. And before it got to the point where I needed to order a mail order brassiere – it would be a cold day in Fort Lauderdale before you'd catch me buying one in the flesh – I resolved to see what my options might be. Because nothing spoils a class reunion quite like having hooters bigger than the prom queen's, and time was running short.

❖ ❖ ❖ ❖ ❖ ❖

Fred was right in his self-diagnosis that he was experiencing the effects of gynecomastia, more commonly known as "man boobs," and more distastefully known in certain circles as *bitch tits*. And he was also right in attributing some of that sudden appearance of flesh above his pectorals to weight gain, even though the source of the weight gain was linked to the source of the gynecomastia, something Fred was about to discover.

With those adjectives, further description of gynecomastia is perhaps unnecessary. The word literally, from the Greek root words that comprise it, means "woman's breast," and there's no mistaking what this means to any man with a shred of masculine self-image. About one-quarter of diagnosed cases cannot be explained (called an *idiopathic* condition, which, by the way, does not mean it happens to idiots), they simply manifest in the course of a man's aging process. Many instances of the condition appear in pre-pubescent or early-pubescent teens, usually when they are over-weight, as well as men in middle age and beyond, both of which suggests hormone imbalances are in play. For teenagers, the condition usually corrects itself as the boy loses body fat and becomes a man over time, but not so for middle age men who suddenly find themselves with a bona fide set of hooters on their hands. The condition can also manifest as a side effect of certain prescription drugs (this comprises about 10 to 20 percent of diagnosed cases) and the diseases that precipitate them, including HIV, kidney and liver disease and other chronic illness.

Less Means More

All that said, the primary culprit where man boobs are concerned is the lack of sufficient testosterone in the man's body. This is intuitively obvious when you consider the great preponderance of cases manifest in teenagers and middle aged men. And even with medical prescriptions that cause gynecomastia as a side effect, those are often the same prescriptions that are designed to reduce the level of testosterone in the body, such as medications intended to treat prostate cancer.

But as you are well aware by now, it isn't just about testosterone. With lowered testosterone comes a proportionately increased level of estrogen (otherwise known as estrogen dominance), and this plays a role in gynecomastia, as well. Because the greater the level of estrogen – women have up to forty times more of it in their bodies than most men – the greater the manifestation of classically feminine physical characteristics.

While the solution to this problem usually involves more than losing a few pounds – although this greatly helps – it also isn't as simple as jacking up one's level of testosterone. Excessively high levels of testosterone can commonly lead to more conversion to estrogen (this is a protective measure), as commonly seen in body-builders who use anabolic steroids. But as Fred is about to find out, most of his problems – including his man boobs – do indeed relate to his level of testosterone, or more appropriately, his lack thereof. And with only a handful of weeks remaining until the reunion, he's about to discover that his options are indeed many, and cause for optimism. Thankfully, none included a surgical breast reduction.

7

Grumpy Old Men

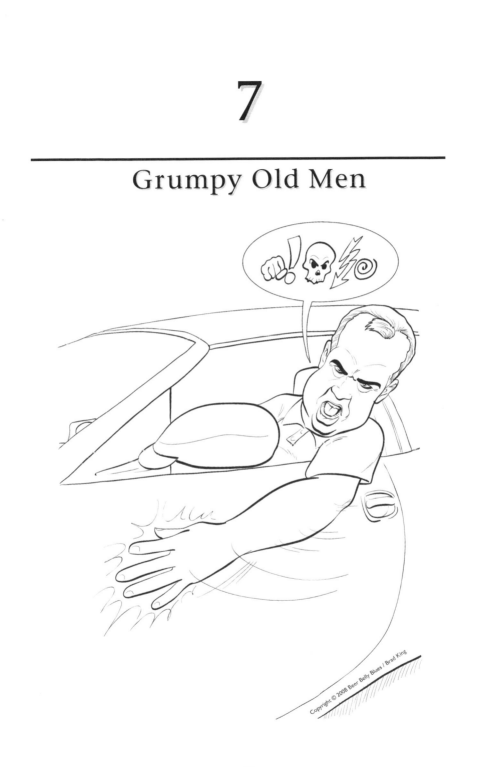

I loved that movie. You remember, the one with Walter Matthau – the M.V.P. of grumpy old men – and Jack Lemon chasing a still-hot Ann Margaret around the neighborhood with pocket-rockets and walking canes. Some guys had fathers upon whom these characters were likely based – I know I did, my father thought the word "goddamn" was in the dictionary, if not the Bible itself – but even then, I doubt that any guy watching, at least anyone under the age of 50, honestly believed they were looking at some Hollywoodized prognostication of their future. So when, during our first ill-fated counseling session, my ex announced to our therapist that I had "lost my love of life and become, in a word, unbearable," and that I had the demeanor of a wounded predator lying on the side of the freeway after a collision with an S.U.V., I was both hurt and surprised.

Of course, my response at the time was something like, "you're a goddamn crazy woman!", thus commencing a full minute of the most awkward silence imaginable. This was followed quickly by a series of equally transparent denials and then, in an attempt to turn the tables – one of my many marital specialties – accusing her of being something woefully short of Ellen Degeneres in the personality department herself, more like Leona Helmsley on P.M.S. When she turned to the therapist and simply said, "See what I mean?" I knew that I was busted, and that she was right: I was officially, even a few years short of my 50th birthday, an utterly impatient, insensitive, insecure, finger-flipping, profanity-slinging grumpy old fart of the first order. With a beer gut, no less.

What I didn't understand about this newly acknowledged truth was the complex relationship between cause and effect that resided at its heart. Was being surly the cause of my present state of mind, which could be described as something along the lines of desperately unhappy, or the effect of a world that had turned on me and was presently plunging knives into my back? On the causal front, I had a bunch of candidates at whose feet I could easily and happily lay the blame, and on the effect end of things, I had to admit that walking through the world with all the positive energy of, well, a wounded animal on the side of the road, wasn't exactly working out, all things considered.

Then again, when you're swimming in the soup – or as my father would call it, the "shit storm," cause and effect doesn't really matter. Either way, you're getting flushed.

And so, as I prepared mind and body for my upcoming reunion, I resolved to manage my inner Walter Matthau for the time being and focus on getting rid of my gut. I could sweat the details of cause and effect later, when I looked like a guy for whom such lofty thoughts might make a difference. Little did I know, I was about to discover that the two – my mood, and my beer belly – had much in common, and in both the cause and effect categories.

❖ ❖ ❖ ❖ ❖ ❖

Poor Fred. At the time he was like that wounded coyote next to the road, lying there without the slightest clue that a veterinary clinic was just around the next bend. Because if he'd have had even the slightest notion that his depression, and indeed, his mood in general, was deeply under the influence of his reduced level of testosterone, and if he'd have had the presence of mind to go to the internet and enter the words "mood," "depression" and "testosterone" into the same search, he'd have been presented with no less than 2,400,000 opinions on the subject. And most of them would be in raging agreement. A man with low testosterone is the equivalent of a grizzly bear that's been woken up prematurely from its winter nap. Either way, someone's gonna get hurt.

Grumpy, or Hormonally Challenged?

But what about the common notion that testosterone causes aggression? After all, aggression isn't exactly conducive to a great mood. Whether you are preparing to play a tennis match or give the big presentation, increased testosterone levels elevate confidence and prepares the mind and body for an upcoming challenge. To date, however, there is no conclusive evidence that directly links testosterone to increased levels of aggression or violence. In fact, our increasingly violent culture has little to no direct correlation with increased testosterone levels. Because of lifestyle factors, collective testosterone levels have been dropping for the past two decades while violence levels have actually increased.

Can you imagine if we've had it wrong all this time? What if instead of using antidepressants like Prozac to treat depression, we actually tried to raise our testosterone levels? What might happen to our mood in that case?

Testosterone and Mood

According to an abundance of research, testosterone has numerous mood lifting abilities. Among its many seemingly miraculous attributes is the fact that it is a great antidepressant. According to one advertisement for a prescription testosterone patch called *Testoderm*, it enhances mood, energy, libido and sexual function. It's interesting how the first mention here relates to *mood*, even above sexual function. According to a study appearing in the *Journal of Clinical and Experimental Endocrinology and Metabolism* that included 856 men aged 50 to 89, depression rates were elevated in nearly direct proportion to falling testosterone levels. The older the subjects tested, the lower their testosterone levels and the higher the incidence of depression. Interestingly, 25 men in the study were already being treated for clinical depression and were on prescription antidepressants. All 25 of these men were found to have the lowest testosterone levels of the entire group, on average 17 percent lower.

In an Australian study of 3,987 older men appearing in the March 2008 issue of the *Archives of General Psychiatry*, researchers revealed a strong link between low testosterone and depression. The study revealed that men who suffered from depression experienced significantly lower testosterone levels than men who had no symptoms of depression. In fact, men with hypogonadism – abnormally low testosterone – are on average 271 percent more likely to show clinically-significant signs of depression than men with higher testosterone levels.

Although it is not known exactly how testosterone enhances mood and reduces depression, it is believed that it works by enhancing a feel-good brain chemical – one that is often low in those suffering from low motivation and depression – called *dopamine*. Another theory is that testosterone aids mood by enhancing energy levels in the brain, and throughout the entire body. Testosterone is actually essential to healthy energy production. In fact, many of the enzymes that manufacture high energy compounds to run our bodies greatly depend upon adequate testosterone for their own production. And finally, there's always that sexy uplifting feeling (called *ego*) a man derives from his muscularity and strength, all of which require gobs of testosterone to maintain as we age.

Life: The Great Equalizer

One interesting aspect of Fred's cause and effect dilemma is that some sources explain depression, and indeed, poor health, away as part of the aging process, exacerbated by lifestyle issues that include level of education, career and family satisfaction, obesity, smoking or other medical conditions. It is interesting to note, with the possible exception of education and career issues, that most of these variables are, in fact, either directly or tangentially related to testosterone. Perhaps this is why patients who don't respond to conventional antidepressants almost always notice an improvement in depression scores when testosterone therapy is administered. The results of these studies, and others, all seem to lead toward the same conclusion: that testosterone is a variable that needs to be embraced and considered in the diagnosis of clinical depression, with testosterone supplementation becoming a viable alternative in many cases.

Of course, when Fred realized he had depression issues he was much more concerned about his belt size. And in fact, when it came to cause and effect, he could easily assume that he was depressed precisely because of how he looked in his pants, or worse, without them. And ironically, in a backdoor-logic sort of way, he would be right. Because when it came time for his naturopathic doctor to check his levels of testosterone, the door would swing open on a discussion that merged both cause and effect into one hopeful course of action, one that just might make his reunion experience even more rewarding than he even dared to hope.

8

The Heart of the Matter

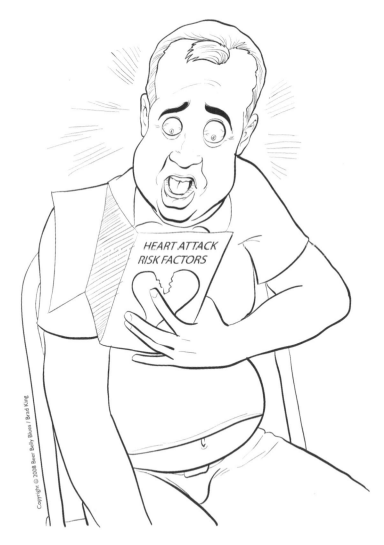

I wish I could blame my ex for breaking my heart. I also wish I could blame her for the turkey gullet under my chin, the varicose veins on my legs that look like a relief map of a lost continent, and of course the escalating price of gas – this was somehow her fault, too – but that's just me. No, my aching heart is another story, and while she certainly gets to sign on as a contributor to its decline in a metaphoric, and dare I say romantic sense, the responsibility for the declining physical state of my ticker belongs strictly to me. I mean, she didn't exactly force-feed all that carbonara sauce down my throat, and for all her nagging about it, the treadmill I bought five years ago still resides in a corner of the garage beneath a pile of unused weather stripping. My bad.

From my point of view, the entire issue of heart health has been reduced to a numbers game. And my numbers have been on a slow and steady decline since my mid-thirties, when I used to brag about my 110 over 60 blood pressure, my 55 beats-per-minute pulse, and my total cholesterol of 185, though I hardly had a clue what any of it meant. I'd watched the numbers begin a ten year ascent worthy of an article in an outdoor magazine, but since none of the differences were particularly dramatic I paid little attention and made few – okay, zero – lifestyle changes to accommodate them. Life is, after all, too short to forgo carbonara sauce.

Then one day I felt something in my chest that reminded me of a playground swing. You know, the ones with the black rubber seats hanging from chains, into which you placed your children and spun them around until they stopped screaming, then stood back and watched them twirl as the chains unwound, assuring them they were having fun all the while. At least until they were throwing up in the car on the way home.

Anyhow, this was what my chest felt like on the day I

discovered the limitations of my health insurance in a big way. Certain I was having a heart attack – this was two years ago, by the way, before my wife began seriously contributing to my level of stress – I rushed to the emergency room (two words: "ten grand") and was immediately plugged into more tubes than Robocop. The bottom line a few hours later was good news – no heart attack – but the bad news was something called angina, which is pain resulting from blockage in the arteries caused by plaque, the biological equivalent of the black grease under your car on the floor of your garage. My doctor wanted to run a tube into my heart through an artery located inches from my family jewels, but given the option to address the problem by making changes to my diet, I elected the latter.

Then began a series of panic diets – I learned quickly how badly I hate the taste of broccoli – and a steady stream of magazine articles clipped by my wife back when she claimed to still love me. Which means, when the articles stopped coming she was suddenly conspiring to kill me, but that's just a theory.

It occurred to me that there might be more to this, however, than one too many hamburgers over the years. I noted with my usual cynicism that heart problems don't appear all that often in younger men, they focus on middle aged and older men, along with all the other assorted benefits of drying up like a human prune during the slow descent to the grave. And the more I learned about the causes of those age-related changes, and the available options to address them, it seemed logical that heart health would also fall into this category of do-not-go-gently-into-that-good-night list of middle age maladies. Maybe, just maybe, it had more to do with the biochemistry of aging than the nature of our diet and the frequency of our exercise, though I had no doubt the latter is directly involved.

The list for my new naturopath was getting longer than the settlement demands from my wife's lawyer. And this one was going straight to the top.

❖❖❖❖❖❖

You may not give it a second thought, but the fact remains that the little muscle in your chest beats, on average, 90,000 times each day, all for the singular purpose of propelling oxygen-infused blood through nearly 100 thousand miles of blood vessels, some of which (called capillaries) are barely wider than the blood cells they are transporting. This biological blood highway can be found in every nook and cranny of your body, which is why a cut anywhere will almost always draw blood. Nutrients and oxygen are moved through the one-cell-thick walls of the capillaries into the fluid that surrounds the cells in your tissues. The capillaries join a network of veins that routes what is now oxygen-*depleted* blood back to your heart, where it is pumped into your lungs to pick up another supply of oxygen. Then the whole process repeats itself – many, many times over every day you are alive – or at least you hope it does. That hope is the very crux of any and all preventative health measures.

But sometimes, even in the best designed systems – and rest assured, our cardiovascular design is nothing short of miraculous – things can go wrong. *Atherosclerosis* is the most common form of heart disease in the developed world. It is characterized by the deposit of cells, usually referred to as plaques, along the walls of arteries. The build-up of arterial plaque can result in narrowing of the arteries, making it increasingly difficult for your heart to do its job due to the restricted blood flow. Researchers have been struggling to unravel the mysteries of heart disease for decades and initially singled out the build-up of cholesterol along artery walls as the deciding factor (among close to 250 possibilities) when calculating the risk of a heart attack. And they were partially right. It turns out that high levels of the so-called *bad* cholesterol, LDL (low density lipoproteins), are only a relatively small part of the problem. Since LDL cholesterol is one of the substances found in those deposits on artery walls, many pharmaceutical companies decided to declare war on LDL, and in the process make a lot of money off a class of drugs called statins. Statins actually block the body's ability to manufacture cholesterol, which means they are a counter-measure against so-called high cholesterol diets. However, further studies over the years have revealed that over half of those who have heart attacks have LDL cholesterol levels that were within the normal range. Obviously, something other than LDL cholesterol is at work here.

It is important to point out that cholesterol also happens to be a major component of cell membranes in all animal tissues, which is why the body deems it important enough to manufacture so much of the stuff (close to 1000 milligrams every day, or the equivalent of four to five eggs). Aside from this important role, cholesterol also happens to be the major building block of sex hormones. And yes, that includes testosterone.

Cholesterol and Testosterone

We happen to live in a world where, if we don't completely understand the role a specific biochemical plays within the body, or worse yet, we can somehow link it to a problem somewhere in the body (in this case our arteries), we can block it altogether just by taking a little pill or two that has been prescribed by a doctor. The problem is that the doctor who is prescribing the medications in the first place doesn't understand the true complications behind taking them. After all, how could they when most doctors take the oath to "first, do no harm" when they enter medical practice?

Choosing to altogether stop the production of one of the body's most important building blocks is a bit like choosing to put all dogs down just because one happened to bite someone. The problem is not so much with LDL cholesterol, but in the overall ratio of LDL to HDL (high density lipoproteins), which is the so-called good cholesterol. HDL happens to be the smallest of the lipoproteins, which is why they are transported within the bloodstream differently than the larger LDL molecules. Because of this size difference, LDL has the potential to contribute to the build up of plaque on artery walls, while smaller HDL molecules actually contribute to its reduction.

Another reason LDL may become part of the arterial plaque buildup is because some studies show that LDL must first be altered or oxidized before it becomes problematic. One example of altering the structure of LDL particles is when you fry or scramble eggs at high temperatures versus poaching or boiling them, which greatly limits the damage to the cholesterol component.

Keeping with this theme, it is also important to have enough antioxidant support in the body (in the form of specialized antioxidant enzymes, fruits and vegetables) to protect cholesterol from damage. The overall ratio of HDL to LDL and the level of antioxident protection in your body is much more important then the total amount of cholesterol found in the blood.

According to numerous studies, low testosterone levels almost always correlate to lower HDL levels and visa versa. Not only are healthy testosterone levels related to healthy (higher) HDL levels, but when testosterone levels are low, HDL is not nearly as efficient at removing plaque from the arteries, and the liver becomes less efficient at removing excess cholesterol from the bloodstream. In other words, in order for HDL to do its job properly, it needs an adequate amount of testosterone to be present.

According to research presented in the 2007 issue of the *Journal of Coronary Artery Disease*, low levels of free testosterone may be related to the development of premature coronary artery disease. The amazing thing about this study was that all the men in the study were under 45 years of age, and yet the results showed that even moderately reduced levels of free testosterone were associated with a 3.3-fold greater risk of developing heart disease compared with men who had normal values. In one of the largest population based studies to date (the Rotterdam Study), researchers looked at the testosterone levels in relation to cardiac health in 504 men aged 67 to 75. The results of the study showed conclusively that the men with the highest levels of free bio-available testosterone had the lowest levels of coronary artery disease.

Endothelial Dysfunction and Testosterone

Many of those who are familiar with cardiovascular problems are still unaware of the term *Endothelial dysfunction*. Endothelial cells are the cells that line the inner surface of all blood vessels, including arteries and veins, making them extremely important to the heart. Endothelial dysfunction is a term used to describe problems associated with the normal function of these cells. Although endothelial cells (collectively called endothelium) have numerous important functions – such as controlling the dilation of blood vessels – when it comes to heart health one of their main functions is to protect the middle blood vessel wall by forming a barrier that prevents harmful substances from entering. Atherosclerosis, or the build-up of plaque within arteries, is now known to occur because of damage to the endothelium (endothelial dysfunction). In other words, atherosclerosis actually occurs when plaque builds up between the endothelium and the middle vessel wall, ultimately reducing the supply of vital oxygen-rich blood to the body's hungry cells.

It turns out that testosterone may play an essential role when it comes to healthy endothelial function. Japanese Researchers from the University of Tokyo recently discovered that men with low levels of testosterone have a much greater risk of endothelial dysfunction. After reviewing hormone levels of 187 men with an average age of 47 who had high cardiovascular risk, the researchers found that those with the lowest free and total testosterone levels experienced the highest degree of endothelial dysfunction.

High Blood Pressure and Testosterone
Medical researchers have known for quite some time that high blood pressure is a major contributor to heart disease. This is a no-brainer. However, exactly how significantly high blood pressure contributes to heart disease has only been speculated, at least until now. After reviewing data from 61 prospective studies involving almost one million people, researchers concluded: "There is overwhelming evidence of a continuous, graded influence of systolic blood pressure, or the peak pressure in the arteries, on cardiovascular disease, morbidity and mortality at all ages." They go on to say,

"It is the level of blood pressure that kills, not arbitrarily defined hypertension. The importance of what appear to be trivial differences in blood pressure, even within the high-normal blood pressure range, should not be underestimated. The extra effort needed to lower the blood pressure down to the recommended goals for avoiding cardiovascular disease is worthwhile."

A ground breaking study appearing in the 2003 journal, *Hypertension*, showed that high blood pressure was intricately linked to low testosterone levels in 119 non-obese, non-diabetic and nonsmoking men aged 60 to 79. The study showed that those with the lowest testosterone levels experienced the highest blood pressure readings.

Metabolism and Testosterone

Finally, testosterone plays a major roll in reducing the incidence of heart disease through its effects on body fat, metabolism and exercise tolerance. Testosterone is required for muscular activity, size and strength, and since muscle is one of the body's critical metabolic engines, common sense would dictate testosterone also reduces heart disease risk by helping the body burn more fat. And everyone understands that excess body fat is not exactly your friend when it comes to optimal heart health.

Constant fatigue and an inability to exercise regularly (poor exercise tolerance) are both side-effects of heart disease. One of the primary reasons people who suffer from cardiovascular problems experience these common side-effects is because they tend to lose a great deal of muscle mass, strength and endurance due to poor heart function. With heart disease, the heart muscle literally loses its ability to manufacture adequate energy in the form of ATP, the body's chief energy substance. According to researchers from the University of Sheffield in the UK, the drastic decline in energy experienced in heart disease may be in large part due to a decline in testosterone levels. The researchers suggest that androgen (testosterone) therapy may be a potential treatment in these instances.

Anyway you look at it, testosterone can no longer be ignored when it comes to healthy heart function. And if our friend Fred goes about it right, because of it he won't be ignored at his high school reunion, either.

9

Stress and Immunity

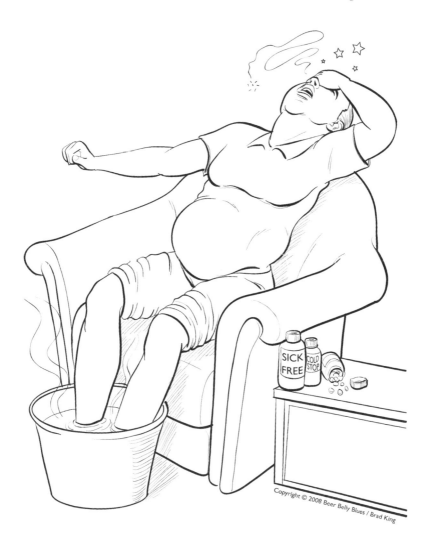

Copyright © 2008 Beer Belly Blues / Brad King

In case you haven't been paying attention, it's not easy being me. I've heard people spew that line for years, and it always sort of disgusted me, as the self-aggrandizing world view of others often do. Because in most cases whatever it was that in their view made it hard to be them was, in fact, a creation of their own construction. But when it comes to the guy looking back at you in the mirror – it's not easy being him, either – that very truth becomes an ironic complication to the very same cliché, the one with my by-line. When you know you're the one who has punched all those holes in the hull of your sinking ship of a life, it makes it just that much harder to deal with both the reality of your situation and the fact that you have no one else to blame. Or at least, no one other than that schmuck looking back at you from the mirror, telling you it's hard to be you.

Such maddeningly paradoxical thoughts are, I've come to realize, a source of great stress in my life. And with my 25-year reunion-inspired push to reinvent myself, I'm looking at all angles of what that means. The only thing I really knew about stress was that it sucks. And now that I'm delving into the dark academia of it all, I don't like what I'm learning. Because while it's usually things like high blood pressure and heart problems and tumors and hemorrhages and diabetes and disease (and too often, not paying attention while driving in the fast lane) that take us out, what most men don't realize is that stress is very often the unacknowledged common thread behind each and every one of those nasty end-games. The primary reason men get old before their time and check out long before they need to, is because of the real "cause" in the fatal cause-and-effect dance of life, that one that doesn't appear on either the death certificate or in the obituary, and that's called stress. And where stress is concerned, perception always equals reality.

Once I figured this out – my wife and my doctor had been telling me for years, but the accepted "man-code" of our society doesn't allow us to respond to such warnings – everything suddenly changed. It was admittedly wonderful to finally have something to blame for all my troubles – stress – which, while perhaps comforting, didn't do a thing to lessen its effects. In fact, I got more stressed-out just thinking about it.

Further study brought an even darker understanding about stress. Because while one can work directly on it with a massage and listening to a little Yanni – the man-code doesn't permit that, either – there's a deeper outcome to stress that, if left unchecked, is a bit like taking your paycheck to the casino. That's the effect of stress and aging on the body's natural immune system. And in the game of life, you really are governed by how strong – or weak – your immune system is.

There was no hiding from the fact that I don't bounce back like I used to, and haven't for the last decade. Not from catching a cold, not from too much work in the yard, not even from a hangover. Definitely *not from a hangover. In fact, I find myself getting sick more frequently than ever, and then staying sick longer than was the case back in the days when I was still able to throw a football without pain. And no, echinacea and annual flu shots don't work. At least not for me. When I got that invitation to my class reunion in the mail, my first thought (okay, my second thought; my first thought was that I had a gut like Alfred Hitchcock) was that I'd probably be feeling lousy that weekend anyhow, such was the frequency of my alone-time with a heating pad and a bottle of Day Quill.*

I have to conclude that this all had something to do with my age, and thus, my body's ability to heal itself. And perhaps, in my body's ability to fight off cold and flu bugs in the first place. I mean, if I can't seem to grow hair back on my head and keep it from growing all over my back like a cheap rug, if I can't walk without limping for a half-hour after getting out of bed, if I no longer have a sexual thought of any kind while lying there before I try, how can I possibly expect to heal a shin-splint like I used to? No, this was middle age, the training camp for an eternity in hell. I had a sneaking suspicion that the same biochemical processes that were affecting all these other issues were also having a lap dance with my immune system.

Little did I know how right that suspicion would prove to be.

❖❖❖❖❖❖

Fred was on to something where his sneaking suspicions were concerned. Because included in the long list of factors – perhaps lurking behind it all – affecting the level of stress in a man's life, aging, and the state of his immune system as it relates to both, is the same hormone that defines, to some extent, his body mass index and weight, his hairline and his ability to summon an erection when he needs one: our old friend, testosterone.

The research, and thus the accepted conventional wisdom, is vague when it comes to testosterone and its supposed role relative to disease in older men. There's no getting around the very obvious and academically discounted fact that older men get sick more often, and to a greater extent, than do younger men, and do so within a specific set of diseases and conditions. There's also no getting around the fact that heart disease is the number one killer throughout North America, and let's not forget how important testosterone is to an aging man's cardiovascular health, not to mention his overall health and energy. Given the proven decrease in free testosterone as men age, the correlation is inescapable. Yet research often creates a mere dotted line between the two, preferring to assign responsibility for disease in older men to other causal factors.

Some suggest this is the effect of the pharmaceutical industry defining and shaping an optimal market for their products. Some of the best selling drugs out there actually decrease testosterone over time, and it certainly wouldn't serve their mission if, in fact, they acknowledged that a higher level of testosterone, had it been there in the first place, may have played a role in the prevention of the condition, or its treatment.

Testosterone and Immunity
No one disputes that the immunity profile of younger men correlates with peak levels of testosterone in their bodies. Not only is it obvious – check how many young men versus older men are in the nearest cancer ward for prostate surgeries – there are clinical studies that prove it. Some do believe, however, that testosterone can have a suppressive effect on a man's immune system, based largely on the fact that men tend to die at a younger age than women. A closer look, however, one supported by a half dozen recent clinical studies, reveals that the correlation in both directions has a more complex story to tell.

Research has shown that the immune system of younger men reacts in a different manner than that of older men, in a phenomenon known as *immunoredistribution*. For example, immune cells may actually be distributed to the skin and subcutaneous tissues (rather than to the gut to combat intestinal viruses) because evolution has driven them there to help fight infection and promote healing of flesh wounds that may be suffered in combat. It makes no difference that the men of today, for the most part, haven't been in a bar fight, much less real combat – the stresses and resultant diseases of today are relatively new in evolutionary terms, and our immune system's DNA has simply not caught up with the times.

What this means is that testosterone is perhaps getting a bum rap where our immune systems are concerned. Studies suggest that testosterone is indeed sending out signals to the immune system to get busy, but the direction the immune system decides to go from there isn't related to testosterone at all, it's driven by other hormones. So it just may be that while testosterone is taking the rap for suppressed immune responsiveness as men age, it's been on the sidelines all along, having already done its job by sending out a call for help, only to watch without recourse while the immune cells head off to the wrong address, one programmed by thousands of years of evolution.

Stress, Cortisol, and Immunity

Stress and the immune system are inextricably linked in men of all ages. But again, one has only to look at our culture to conclude that older men bring a much longer and deeper history of stress to their biological cells, thus creating a measurable immune system differential. Here is where the testosterone factor comes in, because with less of it in an older man's body, they are less able to support an immune system that is sufficient to win the stress-induced battles and vulnerabilities that are a part of modern life. When it comes to your stress response, being stuck in a traffic jam and letting it get to you is pretty much the same as grabbing a sword and rushing the front lines in a medieval battle, only in this case the opponent is in your own mind, if not the car blocking your way.

When your body perceives stress it releases specialized stress hormones (adrenaline and cortisol), as well as neurotransmitters (norepinephrine and dopamine) that help you deal with the stress until it subsides. This response served our ancestors well, since thousands of years ago they actually needed to battle for their lives with a *fight-or-flight* physical response. Even though stress is a necessary part of your body's defense system, the chemicals it produces can wear your body down if they are summoned forth too often.

Even though all stress hormones, when present in excess, have the ability to damage the body, one in particular – coritsol – has the potential to make things very difficult for your body to remain healthy.

Cortisol is best known for its capacity to inhibit the body's ability to lose weight. The more stress you have in your body, the more cortisol your body will produce, and accordingly, the more weight you will gain, especially around and within (the latter being the real killer here) the abdominal area. Research presented in the journal *Diabetes* indicates that abdominal fat can contribute substantially to the regeneration of cortisol, a true example of things going from bad to worse.

Some companies market products that supposedly inhibit the body's ability to produce cortisol, thus enabling a man to better manage his weight. The solution pays little homage to helping him reduce the stress that resides at the heart of the problem (the production of excess cortisol) in the first place, which of course would lessen the demand for their product, thus exposing the marketing-driven rationale for their cortisol focus. After all, the body still requires cortisol to help control stress, but problems arise – especially as it relates to a man's testosterone levels – when too much of the stuff is manufactured.

During stress, cortisol is viewed by the body as more important than other hormones. And since it is produced along the same biochemical pathway (from cholesterol) as your sex hormones, it usually ends up robbing the body of the very substances needed to keep these hormones at healthy levels. For instance, cortisol can easily compete with testosterone, blocking as much as 50 percent of normal volume. Just ask any stressed-out man about the state of his sex drive and the correlation comes front and center. Libido declines precipitously in the face of stress due to diminished testosterone production (also a result of stress), rather than to the stress itself in a more direct sense.

That alone would be significant cause for a major focus on stress, but it gets worse from there. Cortisol also happens to compete with *dehydroepiandrosterone* (DHEA), your anti-aging hormone, which is why people seem to magically age before your eyes when they are under stress for long periods of time. Healthy DHEA levels are also imperative to a healthy immune system. In fact, one of the ways in which immunity (and aging) is measured is by looking at the DHEA-to-cortisol ratio. Whenever cortisol levels are high, there is a corresponding decline in DHEA along with a suppressed immune system.

Aside from immunity, DHEA is also needed to maintain a healthy metabolism (don't forget your immune cells also have their own metabolism). In fact, research at the University of Wisconsin/Madison has shown that derivatives of DHEA help induce thermogenesis (the burning of bodyfat), and therefore may be able to decrease the incidence of obesity. Since one of the most important rolls DHEA holds in the body is in balancing the effects of cortisol, perhaps this is one of the keys to its metabolism-enhancing effects.

The good news is that DHEA levels can be naturally enhanced by altering your mood. Research presented in the journal *Psychoneuroendocrinology* showed that total mood disturbance and perceived stress over time negatively affected the cortisol to DHEA ratio (cortisol went up and DHEA came crashing down). When the test subjects lowered their stress levels through an intervention called "cognitive behavioral stress management," their DHEA (measured as DHEA-S) levels rose in concert with changes to their moods. In another study performed at the Institute of HeartMath in Boulder Creek, California, 30 test subjects using techniques designed to eliminate negative through patterns and promote a positive emotional state showed a 23 percent reduction in cortisol and a 100 percent increase in DHEA/DHEA-S levels.

Stress and the Immune System

As you are now aware, stress – or more accurately, the cortisol that results from it – dampens a man's immune system to a significant degree. Once again, it's easy to notice the level of health and the instance of disease in stressed men versus those with lower levels of stress. Even a newly-commenced heavy exercise program, which is indeed a source of great stress on the body, often accompanies the catching of a cold within the first few days. This is not a coincidence, but rather, the effect of a depressed immune system stemming from an elevated level of stress.

A quick note here - don't use that last statement as yet one more excuse to avoid exercise. Exercise, in total, acts as a great stress reducer (the body is only under stress while the exercise is underway) throughout the day.

Even that morning cup of coffee – in many instances that *pot* of coffee – can deplete an overworked immune system by raising the level of stress hormones to a point at which they exceed the body's natural response, and keeping those levels elevated for many hours. Researchers from Duke University published a study in 2002 showing that stress hormones elevated by daily caffeine consumption – even moderate consumption – caused blood pressure elevations and increases in stress reactivity that could contribute to an increased risk of coronary heart disease in the adult population. Consider the number of people with a coffee habit, this is a sobering revelation.

It is virtually impossible to untangle these stress, cortisol, immunity and testosterone-level variables in assessing the state of a man's health, especially an aging man whose testosterone levels are diminishing. Our evolutionary DNA is what it is, and no amount of debate will change that reality. Only our response to it can change, and the time is at hand.

Kids get colds all the time, yet few experience serious effects and consequences, and even fewer die from them. Yet, over 60,000 adults over the age of 64 die each year from upper respiratory problems and complications arising from colds and flu. Could it be that as we age our immune system is, when alerted, sending its assets to the skin to ward off infection from animal bites and stray arrows, rather than to the lungs to fight off cellular inflammation? Could it be that it is our internal wiring, along with too much stress and not enough testosterone, that is the real culprit in a man's suppressed immune system? The latest research suggests that it is.

As seen with DHEA, there is also a proven correlation between the emotional state of men – specifically, depression and anxiety – and the level of free testosterone in their blood. A proven correlation also exists between depression and compromised immunity to disease. Depressed men get sick more easily, more often, and more severely. Because of this, testosterone suddenly becomes a remedy instead of a scapegoat. As mentioned in Chapter 7, clinical studies have proven that testosterone is a natural anti-depressant, if nothing else for the increased level of energy, muscularity, strength and libido it helps create and maintain. From this it is easy to see how the maintenance of a healthy level of testosterone is a natural and effective avenue of response for men looking to fight off the ravages of stress and depression and the devastating impact those conditions have on their immune systems.

At The Cellular Level

How does this work, biologically-speaking? The presence of natural testosterone promotes the body's ability to repair itself, a process called *anabolism*. In normal metabolisms, there is a balance between testosterone and cortisol, which creates a healthy balance between the body's breakdown (cortisol/catabolism) and repair (testosterone/ anabolism) processes. Stress tips the odds in favor of favor of breakdown, and thus the body has a harder and harder time keeping up with the damage. In reality, premature aging is exactly this process – the body's inability to repair faster than the damage occurs.

By upsetting the natural process of breakdown and repair, stress, in turn, makes us fat because it also contributes to insulin resistance, which invariably puts our body into a fat storage mode (due to the need for excess insulin) and greatly increases our risk of metabolic disorders such as Type 2 diabetes. Aside from this, cortisol also destroys our metabolism by blocking our ability to efficiently synthesize protein to maintain and rebuild muscle, and by now you are well aware of how important muscle is to metabolism.

The bad news is that it isn't just cortisol that wreaks all this havoc – *aging* has the same effect. Why? Because aging comes with a reduction of testosterone, which is necessary to balance the presence of cortisol and other catecholamines. That's right, aging is synonymous with higher cortisol and lower testosterone, not to mention DHEA and all the other valuable hormones we produced in abundance in our younger years.

The conclusion is as clear as it is inescapable: to combat the effects of stress and its relationship to a reduced immune system, not to mention a shifting landscape where prostate health is concerned, a man must take steps to ensure that his testosterone levels remain sufficient as he ages. And because the body has gradually abandoned that mission over time, a man must use other means than his natural, unassisted ability to produce the testosterone he requires.

PART TWO

The Education and Reinvention of Fred

10

We Really Are What - And *How* - We Eat

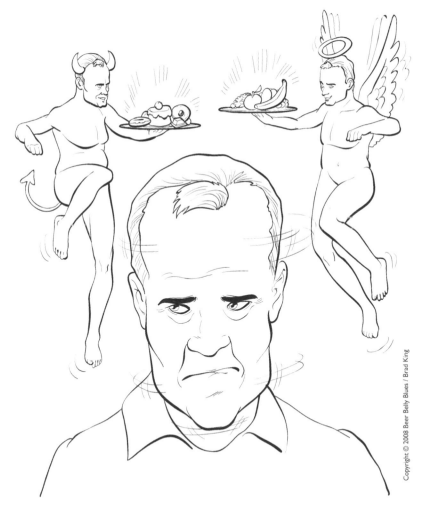

Like many people with too much time on their hands, I used to sit around and wonder what heaven would be like. My version of heaven was a place where you could eat anything you wanted, any time you wanted it, and never gain an ounce. I'm talking wall to wall potato salad and pie. Of course, I'm not the first person to imagine heaven like this – most of them look like Pavarotti – and I won't be the last. Because until someone returns flapping a pair of feathered wings and tells us otherwise, it's hard to imagine anything that would be a better eternal reward.

But this isn't heaven. It's Planet Fred. At least for me it is. Draw your own conclusions about how far from heaven that really is. But I digress...

This little fantasy about a calorie-free heaven is how the term "reality sucks" came into being. Because the reality of eating healthy with a goal of losing weight had been, in my experience, the very essence of hell itself. I was good for about three days, and when I hadn't lost the ten pounds I'd been shooting for in that time, I figured what the hell and went back to fries with tarter sauce.

So I was relieved when my naturopath gave me material to read concerning the real way to lose weight by adopting better eating habits, and it had nothing at all to do with "going on a diet." In fact, it didn't take long for me to sign up for the new conventional wisdom that diets don't work at all. Trying to lose weight with a diet, and then thinking you can keep it off when you go back to all that potato salad and pie, is like trying to repair a leaking dam with spackle and chewing gum. It may last for a while, but sooner or later that dam is gonna burst and the valley will be flooded with deep fried food and a never ending river of ice cream. No, what it takes is knowledge, and the realization that you don't have to starve yourself to reach your body fat goal and stay there.

Hey, I did it, and if I can do it so can you. Listen, it ain't quite heaven (I'm still on Planet Fred, after all), but things are looking up for me. Now if someone would invent some fat-free, calorie-free tartar sauce that doesn't taste like liquid car wax... now that would be heaven.

❖❖❖❖❖❖

The last thing the world needs is another boilerplate white paper on the principles of diet, nutrition and the eternal quest of losing weight, and you're not going to get one here. In fact, rather than a white paper, we can sum it up in a very few short sentences.

Here they are: Eat less. Eat better, smarter, cleaner. Eat more often (five smaller meals, rather than the traditional three). Eat an informed diet that takes your present size, level of activity and goals into consideration. Eat a lot of fiber. Avoid white flour products, starches (such as potatoes), and sugar, because these spike your insulin levels (which we'll cover shortly). Yep, sugar makes you fat, end of story.

That's it. There's an entire bookstore and an internet full of material that expands and expounds on these few sentences, all without really changing them.

Now let's go deeper into one of those short sentences. The one with the words eat *smarter* in it.

What the world *does* need, at least the male half of it, as well as women who want to understand how to better share the cooking and dining experience with that male half, is a better understanding of how your diet can effect your hormones, especially insulin. The good news for those seeking to shed a few pounds is that a hormone-friendly diet is also a fat-unfriendly diet, which means the goals of losing weight and maintaining a healthy level of testosterone well into middle age and beyond are not mutually exclusive. The better news, however, is that a man who understands how the food he puts into his body can have a significant effect on his ability to produce natural testosterone is empowered to change his life in many ways, and not just when it comes to losing weight.

Insulin, the Hormone of Fat Storage

The human body is designed to do one of four things with the foods we consume: 1) burn some of the calories as immediate energy; 2) use the proteins and fatty acids to replace and repair cells; 3) store some of the excess sugars from the diet as short term energy (referred to as glycogen, which are long chains of sugar molecules) within the liver and skeletal muscles; and 4) store any of the left over sugars (once glycogen levels are full) in its 30 billion fat cells.

The average human body only requires about one level teaspoon (5 grams) of blood sugar at any one time to run its millions of biochemical reactions. At the same time, our bodies only have the ability to store about a half days worth of glycogen, which means we have quite the limited storage capacity for sugar.

According to recent statistics from the *Third National Health and Nutrition Examination Survey*, the macronutrient that comprises the majority (50%) of our modern day diets comes from processed carbohydrates. These are also referred to as high-glycemic or fast releasing carbohydrates that break down and release their sugars quickly. By over- consuming the wrong types of carbohydrates (not fruits and vegetables), we generate a rapid increase in blood sugar levels, which in turn causes the pancreas to pump out excessive loads of insulin. Insulin is essentially a storage hormone that not only lowers blood sugar, but also has a powerful message for your fat cells: *store fat now!*

Insulin accomplishes this task by stimulating a very powerful fat storing enzyme (called *lipoprotein lipase*, or LPL) that expands the fat cells, all the while making sure that fat doesn't get used as a fuel source. LPL is so good at its job that many obesity researchers refer to it as the gatekeeper of fat storage.

Since our bodies only have a limited storage capacity for carbohydrates, any carbohydrates not used immediately by the body or stored as glycogen are, with the aid of LPL and of course insulin, converted into triglycerides and stored within the 30 billion fat cells throughout the body. As you can see, a food does not have to contain fat to become fat in your body. No, it's sugar and it's effect on insulin that does this dirty job.

Just as we can set the tone for continual fat storage through wrong dietary choices, such as excess high glycemic carbs, inactivity and excessive stress, we can also create the proper environment for continual fat loss by avoiding fat-storing (processed) carbohydrates and consuming more fruits and vegetables, high quality proteins (including grass fed varieties of beef, game meat when and if available, organic free run chicken, organic eggs, fish and whey protein isolates) and good fats (fish, flaxseed, hemp, almonds, walnuts, etc.).

Good Fats, Bad Fats and Everything in Between
The majority of our planet is obsessed with the bathroom scale. Almost everyone has tried to lose weight at

one time or another, but unfortunately almost no one has asked the right question: "where is the majority of the weight loss — on whatever diet you follow — going to come from?" At first glance this may seem like a silly question. However, once you understand that it is as easy to lose almost as much muscle as it is to lose fat while on an unbalanced fad diet, you quickly come to the realization that perhaps *weight loss* as you know it may not be all it's cracked up to be. After all, you can lose weight by having your gall bladder removed. Losing *weight*, per se, isn't the goal; losing stored *fat* is.

It is critically important to understand your goal when you go on a diet. As mentioned, not all weight is created equal (try telling this to a woman eagerly awaiting the beginning of swimsuit season). No one can afford to lose precious muscle mass – especially if you are in the middle of the Beer Belly Blues – as muscle is the major metabolic engine of the human body, which ultimately dictates to a large extent how many calories you can burn each day. When you lose too much muscle on a diet, which can easily happen on an unbalanced program, you essentially become nothing more than a smaller fat person. So although you might lose weight fast on a fad diet, you may be allowing your muscles to atrophy – think anorexia – which is definitely not a goal you want to embrace. So the better goal is to concentrate on losing *fat*, rather than losing *pounds*. As we've pounded home, there is significant difference between the two. A healthy diet is a significant factor in the fat loss process, and there are certain principles and protocols that make it happen faster and with a higher level of safety than others.

But fat loss is not the only worthy goal, even for those to whom this is the primary concern. Informed dieters know that while calories do indeed count, they are not all created equal, and that there are other biological variables involved in the process. One of the most important of those other variables is testosterone, which regulates the rate at which men gain or lose muscle mass in relation to their nutrition and level of activity. And as we know, muscle mass and its endless pursuit is the best weapon of all against fat. Trying to lose fat without optimizing one's level of testosterone is like trying to make money in a depressed stock market. It can be done, but the enlightened participant understands that certain conditions call for specific measures and protocols that are fine-tuned to optimize the environment at hand.

One of the most common principles of dieting to lose fat is to cut down on high-fat foods, or the common *low fat diet*. Fat, of course, delivers nine calories per gram, whereas carbohydrates and proteins deliver only four. Therefore, or so goes the uninformed logic, the lower the fat intake, the lower the calorie intake, which serves the weight loss goal. However, much research indicates this is not the case.

The problem is that almost all low fat diets are rich in excess carbohydrates and too many carbohydrates – especially the wrong kinds – can place your body in a perpetual fat storage mode. Aside from this, when excess carbohydrates are added to processed food and to your menu choices to replace the flavor component of a reduced fat diet, a significant percentage of the supposedly "saved" calories are back in play, or should we say, back on your plate, and before long, back on your butt. But that isn't the only potential risk of such an approach. A study at Rockefeller University in New York compared test subjects who consumed a 40 percent fat diet (40 percent of total calories in the form of fat) to those on only a 10 percent fat diet. Blood was drawn every ten days for the express purpose of seeing how much fat was present in the bloodstream. Because the body is very good indeed at making it's own fat, and because carbohydrates are, in fact, the raw material of that internal fat-making process (in the form of insulin secreted as a response to the elevated presence of carbohydrates), they found that the high-fat group had virtually no naturally-produced fat (also known as cholesterol, which is giving away the punch line of this story), as measured by triglyceride levels. The group with a low fat intake had an elevated level of naturally-produced fat, because the body, in sensing a deprivation of incoming fat, made up the difference, and then some. In fact, doctors in that study discovered that 30 to 75 percent of the fatty acids present in the blood of this group consisted of saturated fat manufactured in the body.

Back to Our Prehistoric Past

Not all fats are equal in terms of risk and nutritional value. Until relatively recently, mankind existed on a natural diet that was heavy on wild game meats, fish and nuts. These low glycemic foods were rich in the type of friendly fats that helped the body keep "bad cholesterol" levels in check, and kept "good cholesterol" levels where they should be. Today, however, our diet is vastly different than that of our forebears, with an extraordinarily high level of saturated fats and high glycemic carbohydrate calories. The result is an elevated level of unfriendly fat-related diseases, with cardiovascular disease leading the way. This is in addition to obesity, diabetes, hypertension and arthritis, just to name a few whose advent and prevalence in our culture is directly related to our high glycemic diet regimen.

Cholesterol, in the right form and at the right level, is a

good thing indeed. But like so much of our modern way of life, there can be too much of a good thing, and that's were *eating smart* comes into play.

Too Little Too Late

Every cell in the human body depends on cholesterol in order to maintain a healthy and fluid cell membrane (the coating around the cell which allows nutrients in and waste products out). Numerous experiments show conclusively that the health and fluidity of cell membranes change when cholesterol levels get too low. How exactly? Dr. Beatrice Golomb, Professor of Medicine at UCSD, set out to answer the question of what happens when men experience excessively low cholesterol levels. Through her research she discovered that fifty percent of men whose cholesterol levels were below 150 mg/dl had more violent deaths than men with higher readings. In all, Dr. Golomb reviewed 163 studies that connected low cholesterol levels to violence and suicide. The scariest part was that cholesterol-lowering medications were also associated with increased risk of death by violence. From this and other research, it appears that for most men, cholesterol levels below 150 mg/dl can be dangerous.

Testosterone and Cholesterol

Testosterone levels are affected by diet because of a little known yet critically-important facet of nutritional truth: cholesterol is the building block of sex hormones, including testosterone. Which means, when we go out of our way to reduce cholesterol in our bodies, and do so without understanding the consequences as well as the *right* versus *wrong* way to go about it, we pay a price in terms of adequate testosterone production. And as we know by now, the price of that is measured in many ways for men entering middle age and beyond.

One of the problems in making this discussion clear and assessable to the general public is the over-simplification of the concept of cholesterol. We're just now getting our head around the fact that not all fats are evil life-sucking poisons in our bodies, this after decades of belief to the contrary. The same evolution of thought is now at hand when it comes to the issue of cholesterol. Here's the primary misunderstanding that prevails: people think that the cholesterol content in the food we eat (especially eggs, the poster child for high cholesterol food) is the same as the cholesterol in our blood, the stuff that, when it sticks to the walls of our arteries, kills us by the millions. This belief is perpetuated by the pharmaceutical and food companies who benefit from the marketing of low-cholesterol products. Recent studies, however, say otherwise. In fact, they say that there is absolutely no relationship or association between dietary cholesterol – the stuff we consume in our food – and the cholesterol floating around in our collective bloodstream. Two of the most significant long-term studies on this issue, by fellows named Framinghand and Tecumseh, found that there was no difference in blood levels of cholesterol between those who consumed high amounts of dietary cholesterol and those that didn't.

But there were other differences. Those who regularly consumed food rich in *dietary* cholesterol were generally associated with higher muscle mass and strength, with the conclusion that this stemmed from a higher level of testosterone production, as well as enhanced tissue repair capability. Other studies have confirmed that testosterone is an essential element in efficient tissue repair, including muscle cells damaged through resistance training (also known as *weight lifting*). Cholesterol levels in the blood are known to rapidly decrease following intense weight lifting, possibly due to the fact that the body is using them to begin the process of muscle cell repair. The conclusion is that when the body is provided with sufficient blood cholesterol following intense muscular work, it recovers more efficiently. This does not, however, mean you should eat gobs of cholesterol-rich foods after your workout, it simply means that blood cholesterol is essential to muscle recovery.

The conclusion for those seeking to keep their testosterone levels within healthy ranges is inescapable – a low-fat diet is not the ticket. Your body needs essential friendly fats to function as designed, and any deprivation of the intake of those friendly fats compromises that functionality. Now, for those who are concerned about the effect of a high fat diet on heart health, the good news is that the incidence of heart disease in North America has not changed to any degree in spite of consuming a diet that consists of lowered amounts of saturated fats. As long as you don't over do it, eating friendly fats will not harm your health or raise your blood cholesterol levels.

When we think of dietary fat, most of us quickly picture a plate of eggs at the breakfast table. In a recent study published in the 2008 issue of the *Journal of Nutrition*, it was shown that the prevailing fear of getting too much "bad" cholesterol from eating eggs was simply not a valid one. Subjects in that study were given three whole eggs per day (equal to 640 milligrams of dietary cholesterol), or an equivalent amount of a cholesterol-free egg substitute. To the great dismay of the folks marketing their so-called "healthy heart" egg substitute products, the group eating the real eggs showed an elevated level of "good" cholesterol (HDLs), without an associated increase in the level of "bad" cholesterol (LDLs and triglycerides). Since higher levels of HDL are associated with a *reduced* risk of heart attacks, it could be concluded that we should actually be eating more eggs instead of fewer.

Too Much of a Good Thing?

When it comes to dieting, it's generally true that too much of virtually anything is unhealthy, including saturated fat. Like vitamins, minerals, overall calories, and even water, there are ranges and healthy limits to observe, too little or too much of any one can have unhealthy consequences.

Research indicates that moderate fat intake comprising approximately 30 percent of dietary calories, with an emphasis on healthy and non-saturated fats, is the optimal target level for overall health and testosterone production. Consuming too little can raise the body's naturally-produced blood cholesterol to levels that are a cardiac risk, and for those who believe that "more is better," these same studies show that once the optimization level of fat consumption for natural testosterone production has been reached (mainly through eating heart-healthy monounsaturated fats from olive oil, avocados and nuts, especially almonds), consuming more will not elevate testosterone levels even further. The point is not to gorge yourself on fat, but rather, to make sure you are getting enough friendly fats to allow your body to create an optimized environment for testosterone production.

When friendly fat consumption falls below 15 percent of total caloric intake, the risk of experiencing low levels of biologically-active free testosterone in the blood elevates, in addition to depleting the presence of the anti-aging hormone DHEA. DHEA has also been seen at a depleted level in those who have elevated stress hormones, such as cortisol, which also deplete testosterone. Vegetarian diets can run the risk of violating this lower threshold for friendly fat consumption, along with the risk of an elevated SHBG (sex hormone binding globulin) levels, which like low testosterone, is bad news for andropausal men, because it actually compromises testosterone production.

Bottom line: a low-fat diet with a high stress lifestyle can be the worst caloric cocktail of all where testosterone is concerned.

Trans Fats and Testosterone

The vast majority of our processed food – *processing* being another way our diet differs from that of our ancestors – delivers a high level of what is known as "trans fats" into our diet. Trans fats are in actuality hydrogenated plant oils – think Crisco – used in the production, preservation and preparation of food. They normally start out in unsaturated (both poly- and-monounsaturated) liquid form at room temperature, but are made to look like saturated fats with the addition of extra hydrogen atoms (hence the term "hydrogenated"). This hydrogenation process allows the new, partially saturated fat to remain solid at room temperature, as well as demonstrating a higher melting point and longer shelf stability, which is all ideal for products involved with baking. But not so ideal where your health is concerned.

Trans fats are bad news for testosterone. They are, in fact, the worst dietary enemy for those eating with a view toward an optimized testosterone environment in their bodies. High levels of trans fats have been shown to cause a reduction in HDL levels in the blood – not a good thing – while raising LDL levels, an even worse consequence. Not only is this a risky environment for your heart, it's the worst-case scenario where your natural testosterone production is concerned.

Protein and Testosterone

Perhaps as much as testosterone itself, nothing smacks of muscle quite as much as the word *protein*. Proteins are the very building blocks of muscle tissue, and a necessary element of our diets if we are to grow and repair muscle tissue, which all of us must do, even if we've never seen the inside of a weight room. Research shows that a diet rich in protein contributes to greater gains in strength and muscle mass during resistance training in comparison to a diet dominated by high-carbohydrate foods. Not to mention the fact that high-protein foods are more satisfying, fill us up quicker and are often healthier than most high-carbohydrate foods. A couple of questions clarify this statement: which is the more satisfying meal – a bowl of cereal or a steak? A plate of beans or a couple of chicken breasts? Case closed.

Protein-intensive meals (along with high-fat meals) send a satiety signal to the brain in a way that carbohydrate-intensive meals do not (which is why, at least in the folk-lore of the modern diet, you are often hungry an hour after stuffing yourself with Chinese food).

The best source of dietary protein is lean chicken and turkey breasts, fish, seafood, egg whites and whole eggs, and cross-flow microfiltered whey (especially whey rich in alphalactalbumin), as well as leaner cuts of wild game. Other good sources of protein include organic yogurts and cheeses, organic cottage cheese and hemp.

So where's the beef? Beef is certainly a rich source of

protein, but because it is higher in saturated fat content you are likely to reach that 30 percent dietary fat threshold sooner rather than later. These other sources of protein allow you to consume much more before reaching the fat-risk level, and are generally more conducive to a testosterone-friendly biological environment in your body.

But healthy fat intake alone isn't the only game in town when it comes to natural testosterone production. Healthy fat intake, along with higher levels of protein, have been shown to raise testosterone levels by lowering SHBG (sex hormone binding globulin), which is the hormone that makes testosterone unavailable to exert its effect on the body. Research published in the *Journal of Clinical Endorcrinology and Metabolism* showed that elderly men who consumed a diet that was low in protein experienced elevated SHBG levels, and thus decreased testosterone bioactivity.

Two words: eat protein. Lots of protein. And don't sweat the fat issue unless you are violating the upper 30 percent threshold. Balance that with smaller amounts of healthy complex carbohydrates to maintain your level of energy, and get to the gym for a testosterone-smart workout (see the next chapter for the basics on that), and you, like Fred, will be amazed at the way your body will respond.

Almost as if you were going back in time.

Because if there's one thing we know about testosterone in a man, is that *response* is everything. If you eat right, you're well on your way to getting it – and let's be honest, every man wants *it* – well into middle age and beyond.

11

Blood, Sweat and Testosterone: The Secret to Efficient and Effective Exercise

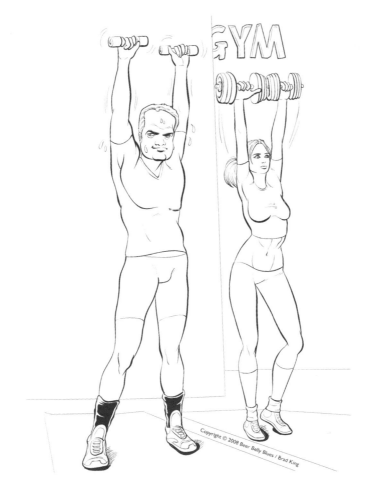

Life is full of humbling experiences. Like your first teenaged kiss, when the girl turns away at the last moment and you stick your tongue in her ear. And then pretend that's what you intended in the first place. Like the time you tried to go through airport security with those Valentine's Day handcuffs (the ones your wife claims she lost) in your carry-on luggage. Or like the time you proudly wore your new suit on your first day at a new job, and just after lunch someone suggested that maybe you should cut the tags off the sleeve.

But nothing says "clueless" quite like your first day in the gym after a 25- year hiatus. Things had changed a bit since my high school days... let's just say I was the only guy wearing tight little nylon running shorts – the shiny kind – that were barely longer than the jockey briefs I wore under them (black, like my socks). I was ready to reinvent myself, just as soon as someone showed me how to use the magnetic card locker key I was handed upon check in.

Who were all these people? Where were all the fat guys like me? Why did all the men over 50 look like they were trying to invent their own exercises? Why were all the guys under 40 lugging around milk jugs full of water – what, the water fountains didn't work? And what was up with all these tattoos of barcodes and Chinese lettering? I would have bet my new Nikes these guys had no idea how to translate their own skin (imagine a tattoo artist with a sense of humor tattooing the words, "I'm a pretentious ass" in Mandarin on someone's biceps while telling them it's the words of Sun Tsu from "Art of War"). I felt like I'd just stepped off the plane in another culture where the language was as foreign as the strange torture devices that lined the walls. At first glance I thought I was looking at farm equipment.

Enter my new personal trainer, the gym equivalent of a seeing eye dog. While I'd like to think I had something to do with the miracle of change that was my body a mere 12 weeks later – I'll take credit for the eating part – the fact is I rarely understood a word she was saying. I just did what she told me to do – risky when you suspect your mentor is secretly a sadist – precisely how she showed me, and arrived on time for each and every session, which at first had all the excitement of a trip to the dentist for a root canal. But then the strangest thing began to happen – the workouts actually started to become fun. Not easy, mind you – no, every time I started to get on top of things my trainer would jack up the weight – but somehow I began to experience a sense of reward and accomplishment. My trainer told me it was my body returning the favor with a little shot of endorphins, and when I thought about it later (usually in the whirlpool, my favorite part of the workout), I think she was on to something there. Because while it feels like work at first, there really is no bigger favor you can do for yourself than pushing it in the gym. Not to the limits of endurance, but to a point where you can feel the biochemical miracle of fat metabolism kicking in. There's nothing quite like knowing all your hard work is bearing fruit, especially when you can eventually see those results in a mirror with your own eyes.

Of course, I hadn't budgeted for a whole new wardrobe as the date of my high school reunion grew near. On the day before the big event, my trainer gave me a hug and wished me well. I told her I'd be back, that there were many more reunions in my future, and that I hoped I wouldn't be going alone next time.

She just smiled and nodded. Then she said the Smithsonian Institution had called about my gym shorts, wondering if I'd care to make a donation to a cultural antiquities exhibit they were developing.

Cute. I told you she was a sadist.

❖❖❖❖❖❖

There's nothing remotely revolutionary about the notion that exercise is good for you, and that it plays an important role in the reduction of a beer belly and the overall improvement of one's health. But now that we understand the effects of aging in men and the unfortunate reduction of natural testosterone that accompanies it, the entire concept of exercise takes on new and even urgent meaning. As important as exercise is in the weight loss discussion, it now stands to play a significant role in the life of men who are experiencing the age-related effects of testosterone loss in other ways. Such as, they look 60, feel 70 and too often behave like they're 80, only they've really just turned 50.

Hold on to your gym shorts, guys, because, there's exciting news for men who want to regain the look and vitality of their youth by boosting their ability to produce and utilize *natural* testosterone in their bodies. And here it is: *exercise.* That's right, the right kind of exercise – with an emphasis on *kind* – plays an important role in natural testosterone production.

The implications of this revelation on the relationship between gyms and male hormones are potentially astounding. If you thought that your time spent at the local fitness center was all about getting back into that tuxedo you haven't worn in years – or worse yet, the dreaded *Speedo* – or even if you have a more evolved sensibility that embraces the management of cholesterol and your general state of cardiac health, now there's another reason to hit the weight room. Because these days we know that certain types of exercise can actually *boost* testosterone production in men, and the benefits of *that* extend not only to the bathroom scale and mirror, but also to the bedroom, the boardroom and even the possible reduction of the need for hair replacement products, or at least hats more suitably worn by guys half your age (hint: nothing says *desperate* quite like a fiftysomething or even a forty-something guy wearing his baseball cap backwards). But before you drop to bang out a quick set of twenty fingertip pushups, you need to understand that, where testosterone production is concerned, not all workouts are alike. Some just make you sweat – always a good thing, by the way – some help make you fit, while others (that also make you sweat) actually *optimize* the body's production of testosterone (among other important hormones), both during and after the workout itself.

It's a nice turnabout, actually – all this time we've been reading about testosterone "causing" muscle growth, usually illegally, when in fact it's really about muscle growth actually *causing* testosterone production. And there's nothing illegal, immoral or desperate about it.

Until recently, conventional wisdom concerning the role of exercise in weight management focused on aerobic activities such as power walking, running, biking or taking thinly disguised aerobic dance classes with your wife that embarrass you into a corner of the gym's padded activity room. And while aerobic exercise remains an important part of a regimen designed to burn calories and improve heart health – hence, the term "cardio" for these exercises, from "cardiovascular" – we now know that the best exercises for testosterone production are done in another part of the building altogether – the weight room. Studies by exercise physiologists such as Dr. William Kraemer (Director of the Human Performance Laboratory at Ball State University), and doctors Fahey, Hakkinen and others, have shown that certain exercises actually contribute to an increase in the body's *production* of testosterone, as a result of the critical mass of the energy required to do these specific, hormone-catalytic moves.

Lifting Weights to Increase Testosterone

The principles of lifting for the purpose of increasing the body's level of testosterone are simple, easy to remember, and totally in harmony with what you already know about the role of resistance exercise in muscle growth and strength. In a nutshell: the greater the resistance on the muscle, the greater the stimulus for testosterone production. And, the more moves you include that involve compound movements and large muscle groups, the more efficient and effective they are with regard to generating an elevated level of testosterone. It's a real-life example of an old adage: the more you put into it, the more you'll get out of it. In this case, the "it" in question is testosterone.

Testosterone and an increase in lean muscle mass go hand in hand, and they occupy *both* ends of the issue of the cause-and-effect continuum: testosterone plays a role in gaining muscle mass (it is the most powerful anabolic steroid there is, and when it's produced by your own body it's not only legal, it's completely healthy), and then once you have all that muscle, your body more easily produces an elevated level of testosterone, if nothing else because of its ability to lift weights in the optimal way that promotes it. Muscles are comprised of tiny fibers which are actually proteins (*actin* and *myosin*). These protein molecules contain nitrogen, which we obtain from food, and also when we break down muscles during work (called catabolic activity). When we increase the retention of nitrogen in the body, the presence of testosterone in turn enhances protein synthesis, or the uptake of protein from food, to repair and build tissues broken down during exercise, which in turn decreases fat and lessens the body's propensity to store energy as fat. When you do this over time it creates a wonderful spiral effect, each level of benefit yielding more easily to the achievement of the next.

How Much is Enough?

In a ground-breaking study appearing in the *Journal of Strength and Conditioning Research* in 1996, men who were experienced weight lifters were evaluated according to the levels of testosterone, serum growth hormone and cortisol (which is detrimental to testosterone and fat loss, and increases in proportion to the level of stress) in their blood using different exercise regimens. One group was put through a routine consisting of one heavy set of a given exercise, while another performed three sets of that exercise, with one minute of rest between sets. Exercises included the leg press, bench press, wide grip lat pull down, shoulder press, seated row, arm curl, leg extension and sit ups, generally a killer whole-body workout. Their blood was drawn before their set(s), then after the routine at 5, 15, 30 and 60 minute intervals.

In both groups, testosterone levels were at their highest immediately following the workout. But the three-set group had significantly higher levels than the men doing a single-set workout, by as much as 20 percent. After 60 minutes, the three-set group again had a *higher* level of testosterone (about 10 percent) than the single set group. Which means, more sets (within reason) generate a greater testosterone yield. Results were even more dramatic where growth hormone was concerned, with the three-set group testing at more than double the post-workout levels of HGH than the one-set group.

The Cortisol-Testosterone Connection

Since weight training is, by design, a stress-inducing activity, post-workout levels of cortisol were also elevated for both groups. It is important to understand, however, the difference between testosterone, which causes protein synthesis, and cortisol, which causes protein degradation. In a post-workout environment, it is critical to have a higher level of protein synthesis than protein degradation caused by excess cortisol, and the way that happens is through the presence of testosterone. With a higher level of testosterone present in the three-set group, which yields a higher ratio of testosterone to cortisol, the effect is enhanced muscle growth, which in turn leads to more efficient weight loss and a long list of other benefits.

The bottom line is easy to get your mind around – for optimal testosterone production through exercise, do three strong sets using compound movements (like squats and dead lifts) that involve more than one muscle group, use heavier weights (but not so heavy that you can't do more than eight repetitions, and not so light that you can easily do more than twelve), and focus on the larger muscle groups. Further studies have evolved this theory to show that even exercises that have always been thought of as heavy – such as the bench press, which doesn't utilize multiple muscle groups other than the pectorals, shoulders and triceps – are not as effective in a hormone-generating sense as are squats, bent rows and dead lifts, which involve virtually the entire body (one of the reasons an exercise like squats can actually help build bigger biceps).

If you workout this way over time, making sure to include a base of heavy, multiple-major-muscle-group lifts in your routine, you'll be creating an optimal environment within your body for increased testosterone production, and all the benefits that come with it.

Interval Training for Increased HGH

The best, most efficient workouts combine resistance exercise (weight lifting) with cardiovascular work (aerobic activities). But as with weight lifting, there is a specific approach that creates an enhanced benefit where calorie burning and weight loss are concerned, and again, it has to do with how it causes the body to produce hormones. In this case, the hormone is HGH – Human Growth Hormone.

Don't let the name fool you. Though one of human growth hormone's key roles in your body is to regulate growth, especially at puberty, its primary role goes far beyond that. HGH is also responsible for increasing lean body mass (muscle) and decreasing stored body fat by freeing it up as an energy source. Don't forget that as we age we lose our vital muscle tissue and gain fat (like we had to remind you of this scenario yet again).

In a landmark study published in the *American Journal of Cardiology*, aerobic training was compared to aerobic with resistance (weight) training. Two groups had to complete a 10-week exercise program of 75 minutes. One group completed 75 minutes of aerobic exercise twice a week, while the other completed 40 minutes of aerobics plus 35 minutes of weight training. The time spent training was identical. At the end of the study, the aerobics group showed an 11% increase in endurance, but no increase in their strength. The group that completed the combination of aerobics plus weight training showed a massive 109% increase in their endurance, and a

21–43% increase in their overall strength. There are many other studies that further prove the theory that resistance training combined with cardio is superior to either one alone.

The technique to optimize the production of HGH through exercise is called "interval training," which delivers the benefit of elevated HGH levels in the body long after you've left the gym for the day, and much longer than a level-intensity aerobic workout. With interval training, even after your heart rate has returned to normal, your body will remain in an elevated state of HGH production for hours.

The best way to visualize this is to picture two types of track athletes in your mind – sprinters and distance runners. Sprinters are built like NFL running backs (and for the very same reasons), with low body fat and thick, powerful muscularity. This muscle mass doesn't slow them down a bit, in fact it is the thing that gives them their explosive speed out of the blocks and the ability to keep accelerating through the course of a race, or a fourth-and-long situation. They burn through their fuel reserves in much the same way a rocket consumes fuel on take-off – it doesn't last long, but it's spectacular while it does, and the effects are the seeming defiance of gravity and physics through power and speed. Distance runners, on the other hand, have bodies that have shed as much muscle mass and fat as possible to allow their bodies to consume fewer calories during a race and thus keep going longer. They are lean, almost to the point of appearing anorexic. The differences in these two body-types is the product of their training – the sprinter uses interval training, while the distance athlete trains using long, low level-intensity work. The elevated levels of HGH and testosterone in the sprinter promote muscle mass, while the demand for calories in the marathoner with a lower level of HGH and testosterone actually discourages the gaining of mass.

The hormonal science that creates the visual differences in these two body types stems from the fact that short bursts of high-intensity work – much like weight lifting – causes the body to produce both testosterone and HGH, both of which promote lean mass and fight the buildup of fat. And like the test subjects discussed earlier, those elevated levels of hormones remain in the body long after the workout, sometimes hours longer after an interval workout compared to a low level-intensity workout. The result of heightened levels of HGH and testosterone is nothing short of the very reason you're in the gym in the first place, because calorie burning is enhanced for hours after the workout and thus the weight management benefits are multiplied, along with all the other benefits of an increase in HGH and testosterone in a man's body.

The key to an effective interval (cardio) workout seems to be doing an activity (like sprinting) for durations as short as 10 minutes in total. You can easily implant this type of a workout at the end of a weight-training routine or on opposite days (i.e. one day weight training and the next interval training). An example of a high-intensity interval workout — using a 5-minute warm up and cool down period — could consist of sprinting on a treadmill full out for 1-minute and walking for the next minute, and repeating this process five times, for a total of 10-minutes of interval work). It is very important to get your heart rate up when you are interval training, so make sure you get clearance from your doctor before beginning this (or any) kind of exercise routine.

Resistance and interval training with testosterone in mind is a powerful tool in the on-going challenge of keeping your testosterone at healthy levels. When combined with a dietary regimen that promotes an optimal hormone environment in the body, along with supplementation designed to help aging men safely maintain the strength, vitality, virility and positive energy of their youth, the path is clear toward a long and productive life that seems to defy time itself.

What to Eat Before Working Out

As mentioned, exercise is stressful on the body, which is why it responds by elevating certain stress hormones such as cortisol. When the body is stressed it isn't interested in digesting food. Instead, most of the blood supply is escorted to the extremities instead of the stomach. This is why you should not consume a lot of solid food *before* exercise, as it will just sit there fermenting in your gut. Instead, you should train yourself to exercise on an empty stomach, or only consume a small amount of calories (try to keep it under 200) anywhere from 30 to 45 minutes before the activity. Contrary to popular belief, carbohydrates are not the best things to eat just before training, since they'll raise your insulin levels, causing you to use glucose (sugar) as your primary fuel.

Instead, the best thing to consume before exercise is protein in a highly digestible form. Protein isolates coming from whey (see Appendix II for recommendations), not only empty from the stomach quickly, but they also cause a rise in the hormone glucagon (the primary hormone for controlling glucose levels during exercise), which allows for optimal fat-burning instead of storage.

What to Eat After Exercise

After any athletic activity, especially weight training, the body requires refueling of its glycogen (stored sugar in liver and muscles) reserves. In order to ensure this happens, the body contains an enzyme called *glycogen synthetase* that is responsible for storing sugar for future needs. Within a 45-minute window after exercise, this enzyme is extra hungry. This is the only time that you can consume larger-than-normal (and higher glycemic) amounts of carbohydrates without worrying that they'll convert to fat. Many of us usually make the mistake of consuming only carbohydrates at this time (fruit juice, for example). This is all wrong, since drinking carbohydrate beverages without sufficient protein after exercise will cause a drastic increase in insulin levels, bringing the increase in growth hormone and testosterone levels to a halt. Recent research confirms that protein mixed with carbohydrates after training allows for faster muscle recovery and greater growth hormone and testosterone increases. Always mix protein with carbohydrates in a liquid form, and do it as close to completing your workout as possible to ensure rapid replacement of bodily sugars and protein for recovery. A good rule to follow is a mixture of between 2:1 to a maximum of 4:1 carbohydrates to protein. The post-workout protein should be primarily in the form of a high alpha-lactalbumin whey protein isolate (see Appendix II for recommendations) for maximum timing and absorption value. The carbohydrates should come from mixed whole fruits, primarily from the berry family due to their superior antioxidant qualities.

Never Underestimate Your Need for Water

It's imperative to increase your water intake during exercise due to its vital role in cardiovascular function and temperature regulation. As you exercise, your body loses a great deal of water through sweating and evaporation, and your muscles create a lot of extra heat. The heat is transported through tiny blood vessels (capillaries) near the surface of your skin. The release of perspiration from your sweat glands and its evaporation from the surface of the skin creates a cooling effect, both to the skin and the blood in the capillaries beneath it. Because of this, sweating is an essential part of your body's cooling system, and it depends on an adequate supply of water to get the job done.

If your body does not have enough water to make this biological cooling system run smoothly, your blood-transporting capacity also diminishes. Don't forget, it is the blood's role to carry nutrients such as oxygen, glucose, fatty acids and proteins to the muscles to create energy. The blood must also remove the toxic compounds of metabolism, such as carbon dioxide and lactic acid. Since your circulatory system is almost 70% water, the extra demand on it can be quite severe. Intensive exercise can cause a 5–8 pound loss of fluid through perspiration, evaporation and exhalation. Studies show that for every pound of fluid lost, there is a significant drop in the efficiency with which the body produces energy. In one study, a 4% loss of body weight from exercise-induced dehydration resulted in 31% shorter muscle endurance time. It's amazing to think that something as simple as water can be the determining factor in winning or losing a competition. Many studies also point out the importance of proper hydration in managing the oxidative stress load of exercise due to the overproduction of nasty little chemicals called free radicals. Still other research indicates proper hydration is essential in protecting and modulating our immune response to exercise.

12

Ultimate Nutrients for the Ultimate Male

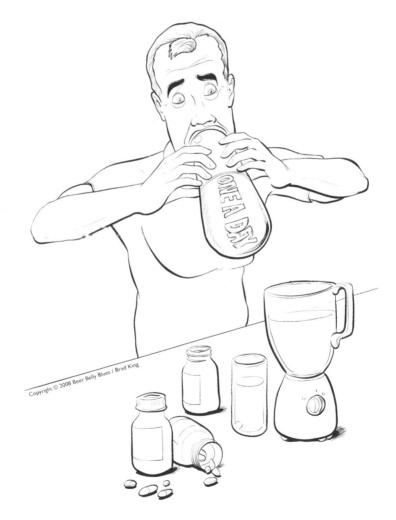

Copyright © 2008 Beer Belly Blues / Brad King

Okay, I was ready for a little intense time in the gym and the sadistic trainer who looked like a supermodel (a strategy for getting fit that I highly recommend, by the way), and I was ready for a complete overhaul to my eating preferences (I was, I must admit, quite happy to hear that I got to eat five or six meals a day). All of that stuff made sense. What I wasn't ready for were all the pills.

No, not diet pills, and not bodybuilding supplements. And not always pills, I was swallowing a few strange roots and berries, as well. Because concurrent with my new exercise and eating plan my naturopath had started me on a regimen of nutritional supplements that were intended, in her words, to "optimize the body's capacity to produce a higher level of natural testosterone." Now, I'd known a couple of guys who were on medically-supervised testosterone – one word: shots, self-administered right where it counts – and it wasn't something I wanted for myself. So I was pleased when my doctor explained that there are several natural herbs and substances that help the body do the job on its own, and that I would be eating them on a regular basis.

Frankly, I hadn't heard of most of them and couldn't pronounce any of them. And I was skeptical at first, especially when my questions about "how" they worked was met with a blank stare and the assurance that "they just do." Then she asked if I needed to understand "how" an airplane got off the ground before I boarded one, and I told her she had a point, because I had no clue there, either, and short of a few weather delays things had been working out just fine.

But it's the strangest thing. After 12 weeks I'd lost a ton of weight, and it would have been easy to give the credit to the workouts and all the nutritious food I'd been eating with surprisingly little sense of deprivation. But the fact is, I knew it was something else. It was the supplements. Not by themselves, but because of the way they were enabling my body to respond to the work and the nutrients. The supplements, when taken with a program of exercise and solid nutrition, became a sum in excess of the parts. My naturopath explained that it's like painting a house without repairing the dry rot underneath... before long after the new paint reveals itself as a temporary fix and you're back where you started. If you deal with the infrastructure – in human terms, the body's natural bio-chemistry and hormone-producing processes – then the work you put in will endure.

So these days it's a new me, both inside and out. And where the inside is concerned, I have those roots and berries and herbs to thank for it. Even if I still can't pronounce their names.

❖ ❖ ❖ ❖ ❖ ❖

There are more folks taking nutritional supplements than anyone realizes. In fact, in most modern cultures more people take them than don't. And they take them for the same reasons some people take the rarer and more exotic supplements, the ones you don't find in the corner grocery store. Because it's virtually impossible to get everything we require in the name of nutrition from food. At least nowadays it is.

The most common – and indeed, the *best* – supplement available today is the common multi-vitamin pill. While purists may argue that nutrition is always best when taken in natural form (this is often true because of the issue of bio-availability, which we'll discuss soon), the fact is that getting all the vitamins and minerals we require for optimal nutrition through natural food sources is just not practical or even realistic. With the advent of processed foods and the hectic lifestyle of today's busy adults (which demands fast and easy eating), trace elements from the list of nutritional requirements are lacking. According to the *Journal of the American College of Nutrition*, the nutritional value of fruits and vegetables in the average American diet has reduced significantly since the 1950s. In fact, only about 19 percent of Americans ingest the daily minimum of magnesium. The problem is so severe that the U.S. Academy of Sciences estimates that adding calcium and magnesium to the public water supply would save up to 150,000 thousand lives annually, most of them cardiovascular-related. And because that's not likely, we need to turn to other means to keep ourselves healthy in this regard. And even if we could, we don't need to overhaul the infrastructure of our society to solve this problem. The best way to get the vitamins and minerals we require for optimal health, and the easiest, is to take a high-quality daily multi-vitamin supplement.

An entire industry has been built around the vitamin niche, and it offers a lot of options. Sure, there are inexpensive brands out there, ones that include your garden variety of inexpensive ingredients. But in this day and age of advanced nutritional science, "cheap" more often than not means you get what you pay for. In this case, when you go the cheap route, what you get is poor results. Always look at the labels to determine quality and quantity of the various substances and their relationship to recommended daily minimum requirements (called RDAs).

Speaking of RDAs – they are fine if you have the metabolism of a sloth. Research, however, is now showing that various nutrients, such as certain B vitamins and vitamin D, need to be taken in higher quantities and in forms that are best utilized by our biochemistry. In this case *optimal daily allowances* (ODAs) are quickly becoming the standard.

Beyond Vitamins and Minerals
The Testosterone Connection

The following nutrients are some of the best choices when it comes to optimizing a man's natural health program and working towards maintaining healthy testosterone production. They are listed last in this section for a reason, because there are no silver bullets when it comes to maintaining an optimal health profile with adequate testosterone levels. The key is to incorporate *all* the various areas discussed in this book, with a healthy diet and exercise program leading the way. Supplements can be an incredible addition – and often the missing element – to a well-designed testosterone-optimizing program, but they are called *supplements* for a reason: because they are intended to *supplement* a well-designed *program,* not substitute for it. They are not nearly as effective when consumed on their own, just as exercise on its own is not nearly as effective as when combined with an effective program of nutrition and sufficient rest. The take-away message here is simple: a synergistic approach is always the best medicine when it comes to restoring an optimal health profile—especially where testosterone is concerned.

Whey Protein Isolate

Due to the numerous complications associated with andropause, men are experiencing serious conditions, including loss of bone density, muscle loss, and increased risk of prostate cancer at younger and younger ages. Recent research indicates that *whey* protein may help combat the symptoms of andropause naturally while promoting better overall health as well.

We already know that protein is good for us, but whey protein is a like a *supercharged* version that many studies suggest can help maintain lean body mass and protect us from harmful toxins. *Glutathione* is an antioxidant that both protects against cell damage while removing powerful toxins from the body like heavy metals and even cancer-causing carcinogens. Glutathione levels are also closely related to overall health and longevity. In animal studies, whey protein significantly boosted glutathione levels more than any other known protein, including soy. This is perhaps why whey protein has also been proven effective in fighting cancer growth, including hormone-responsive cancer cells responsible for breast and prostate cancer.

In one clinical study, patients with varying forms of cancer were given just 30 grams of whey protein versus a placebo group. Those given the whey protein showed signs of regression in more of the various forms of cancer versus the placebo group. A more compelling study involved rats who were fed whey protein (along with a placebo group and groups fed other types of protein) before being purposely exposed to a strong cancer-causing agent. The rats fed whey protein mounted a more aggressive defense against the carcinogen and any tumors produced were smaller and less frequent than in the rats in the placebo group or fed other proteins. A follow-up study confirmed the results and concluded that whey protein offered "considerable" protection against tumors and cancer cell growth.

More research is being conducted to find out precisely

how whey protein helps repel cancer growth but its effectiveness in studies against hormone responsive cancer cells make it a useful tool in the fight to maintain prostate health.

Another major problem caused by lower testosterone levels is loss of bone density and strength. As testosterone levels continue to drop as we age, the risk for osteoporosis increases, but whey protein may be able to help. Animal studies show that whey protein helps improve bone health and overall strength. More research is needed to understand how but researchers believe whey protein stimulates the activity of osteoblasts, the basic building blocks of bone.

Finally, a general loss of muscle mass, tone and strength are also symptoms of both andropause and simply getting old. While lower testosterone levels will make it harder for the body to build lean muscle mass and maintain strength, the loss of protein will produce similar results, which is where whey protein can help.

As the body ages, it becomes more difficult for it to absorb protein, which can lead to a number of issues, including lowered immunity, slower healing times, and the loss of muscle mass. Some proteins, like casein, are absorbed slowly by the body while others, like whey, are absorbed rapidly. In one study conducted by researchers in Europe on elderly men comparing the absorption of slowly digested proteins versus rapidly-absorbed ones, participants absorbed more whey compared to other proteins like casein. While more research is needed to understand precisely why, whey protein helps prevent muscle loss and strength as men age due to poor protein absorption, and may help reduce the loss of muscle mass due to lower testosterone levels.

The research is clear - properly processed whey protein formulas are able to help combat symptoms of andropause, such as maintaining prostate health, reducing cancer risk, reversing muscle loss and reduced bone strength. But on top of helping combat these common and sometimes deadly andropause symptoms, whey protein also appears to dramatically improve overall longevity, at least if animal studies are any indication. In a six-month study conducted on rats who (in human terms) were aged from 55 to 80, an all-whey protein diet significantly enhanced survival rates while improving the overall health of heart and liver tissue.

While it seems that more health benefits of whey protein are being discovered every day, one thing is abundantly clear: for men looking to combat symptoms of andropause and improve overall health, including whey protein in their daily diet is a win-win situation.

Maca

Two troublesome symptoms of male andropause and the lower testosterone levels it causes include a decrease in libido and increased problems with erectile dysfunction. Although cause for concern, these symptoms are by no means unavoidable. Men *do* have safe, all-natural options when it comes to treating them, including a Peruvian root by the name of *Maca*.

The Peruvian maca plant grows only in certain areas of Peru where the mountains are over 13,000 feet high. This plant likes the cold climate and thrives on the thin mountain air and harsh environment. The edible roots look like a bunch of giant carrots, and the people of Peru have been eating them for centuries to enhance fertility and sexual performance in both sexes.   Local traditions also claim that maca is useful in alleviating menopause symptoms (not some-thing too many men will have to worry about) but the root has only recently caught the attention of the medical community.

Animal research bears this out. In a major study using mice, an oral extract of maca root produced significant results, including:

- ❖ Increased Sexual Performance: the maca extract increased the number of complete copulations in test subjects in a 3-hour span versus the placebo group.

- ❖ Decreased Problems with Erectile Dysfunction: male mice with erectile dysfunction that were given maca extract recovered faster between copulations versus a placebo group.

Another rodent study showed that maca improved blood testosterone levels in male mice while also elevating the blood progesterone levels in female mice. This may account for the increased sexual performance and fertility reports in traditional cultures that have used maca for centuries for these very purposes.

In addition to its ability to positively affect sexual performance, maca has also shown great promise in helping reduce problems associated with osteoporosis. Osteoporosis and weaker bones are exacerbated by lower testosterone levels. Chinese researchers discovered that maca was able to improve bone density while strengthening the vertebrae in the back. Researchers don't yet know precisely how maca affects bone density but the root shows great promise in the treatment and prevention of osteoporosis for both men and women.

Finally, maca has even been shown to significantly reduce prostate size in rats. Again, researchers do not know precisely how maca affected prostate size, but it does somehow affect androgen receptors in the prostate, and more research is underway to understand why.

Does it work on humans? According to hundreds of years of anecdotal evidence and a few recent studies, the answer clearly points to the affirmative. In one study, researchers from the University of Peru reported that male sexual desire increased after only 8 to 12 weeks of a daily dose of maca. The amazing thing was that some of the participants only received 1,500 mg of maca, which is equivalent to just two (750 mg) capsules per day. The precise mechanism in maca that enhances sexual desire was not determined but the amazing thing was that serum testosterone levels remained unchanged.

Another four-month human study produced more tangible and startling results for subjects taking maca, including increased sperm count per ejaculation, increased sperm motility, and an increase in seminal volume. Similar results were seen in previous studies and the conclusion is obvious: maca indeed enhances sexual performance in just about every conceivable manner. The next question is, how?

What confuses researchers about maca and its affect on male sexual behavior and performance is that it does not affect overall testosterone levels, at least not directly. In fact, maca does not seem to have a direct impact upon any of the hormones typically associated with sexual stimulation, desire or performance, including testosterone, lutenizing hormone, follicle stimulating hormone, prolactin and estradiol. While testosterone and other sex hormone levels remain directly unaffected by maca, there are two theories pointing to an indirect link. First, it is speculated that Maca enhances bio-available testosterone levels (testosterone not bound by SHBG and thus free for use by the body). And, it is believed that Maca may enhance testosterone receptor binding. Because of testosterone's known affects upon libido, erectile function, and overall sexual desire, researchers appear certain that maca somehow reacts with and/or enhances the effects of existing testosterone levels while not actually elevating them.

But no matter how it works, the results are clear: Maca root helps combat andropause by naturally enhancing sexual desire, improving performance, and reducing problems with erectile dysfunction.

Tongkat Ali

Loss of libido is a major concern for millions of men, and is caused primarily by lower testosterone levels which begin dropping during a man's mid-to late-20's. The question is whether or not there are any natural ways to enhance sexual interest by naturally elevating testosterone levels. And no, we're not talking about Viagra®, as drugs like Viagra® only target the male plumbing but do nothing to positively affect testosterone levels.

For over 1,000 years, Asians have used a plant known as *Tongkat ali* (also known as eurycoma longifolia) as a natural aphrodisiac, and to treat a number of conditions such as malaria, ulcers and low energy (any of which would ruin the sex drive of just about everybody). Researchers have only recently started to discover the true benefits of Tongkat ali, and more research is needed before all the evidence is in. However, the results are very encouraging for this plant being a true aphrodisiac and a natural testosterone enhancer.

Tongat Ali and Male Libido

To illustrate how Tongkat ali affects the male libido, let's look at the libido of adult rats (a parallel more than one woman has made over time). Rats, it seems, are more like humans than we care to admit because they, too, can suffer from a lagging libido. In one study using a special breed of male rats (called "non-copulators" – not the ones who weren't getting any – but rather, the ones who didn't even want any), Tongkat ali was able to significantly enhance mating activities and sexual initiation versus the placebo group.

Thankfully, most of us don't consider ourselves non-copulators, so another study decided to focus on how Tongkat ali affected normal everyday sexual experienced rats. After determining what constituted as normal sexual activity (could you imagine being the researcher who had to define this?), the researchers discovered that Tongkat ali significantly affected what they called "mounting behavior." That's right, the higher the dose of Tongkat ali, the *hornier* the rats became, as evidenced by their increased attempts at mounting and initiating sexual intercourse. One study even concluded that Tongkat ali enhanced the libido in inexperienced, castrated rats (a contradiction in terms if ever there was one).

Tongat Ali and Testosterone

Testosterone is known to help increase fat-free mass, muscle mass and overall muscle strength, and recent studies indicate that taking Tongkat ali produces the same effects. In a double-blind study reported by the *British Journal of Sports Medicine*, subjects taking Tongkat ali for five weeks and undergoing brief but intense strength training showed dramatic results, including:

* ❖ 5% increase in lean muscle mass
* ❖ increased fat free mass
* ❖ reduced fat
* ❖ increase in muscle size and strength

These are the exact same results you would expect from taking a testosterone treatment, but the only thing the participants received was Tongkat ali. The participants receiving the placebo also underwent the same intense strength training but showed no significant improvements in any of the areas listed. Unfortunately, this study did not measure free testosterone levels, though the results certainly indicate Tongkat ali produced testosterone-like effects in the test subjects.

One researcher at the Human Reproduction Specialist Centre in Malaysia (Dr. Tambi) conducted a study on 30 healthy men (humans this time), looking at the effects of Tongkat ali on virility. For three weeks the men were given Tongkat ali, and the results were amazing because not only was this incredible plant able to enhance virility, but testosterone levels had doubled in just three weeks.

Because Tongkat ali is relatively new to western science, most studies on this plant are from Asian nations like Malaysia. So while the testosterone levels doubled in the test subjects in Dr. Tambi's study, further research is needed to fully understand precisely how Tongkat ali affects testosterone levels and to what extent. Another larger study by Dr. Tambi, this one with government backing, is currently underway involving 200 subjects.

The most convenient and practical way to include Tongkat ali in your daily diet is to consume it in supplement form in a 100:1 extract, the same ratio that was used in the studies. Be sure to look for all-natural Tongkat ali supplements because synthetic ingredients are harder for the body to recognize and use because they have lower bio-availability).

Chrysin

One of the largest "natural" threats to testosterone levels in men is due to a conversion of testosterone to estrogen via the *aromatase enzyme*. This is every body builder's worst nightmare (two words: man boobs), and it is something than anyone working with their testosterone level needs to be aware of. Because it's preventable, but only if you understand the chemistry behind it.

A naturally occurring enzyme concentrated primarily in belly fat (abdominal fat cells) and skin of the scrotum, aromatase converts testosterone and other androgens into estrogens. Basically, testosterone levels decrease naturally as men age because aromatase is converting the primary male sex hormone into the primary female sex hormone, estrogen. Two factors known to increase aromatase activity are poor nutrition and high levels of belly fat, which means, in essence, that the fat get fatter. Research indicates that increased levels of physical activity and eliminating abdominal fat can naturally lower aromatase activity and thus help maintain higher testosterone levels. Aside from the obvious — physical exercise and getting rid of the old beer belly — nature has provided men with a natural way to reduce aromatase activity, and in the process help avoid the medical problems associated with lower testosterone levels. It's a substance called *chrysin*, and it's one of nature's most potent and best aromatase inhibitors.

In vitro (test tube) studies consistently reveal that chrysin effectively inhibits the aromatization of both testosterone and androstenedione. Research has shown that chrysin also forms weak bonds with alpha and beta estrogen receptors, further helping men limit estrogen levels while maintaining testosterone levels.

The majority of evidence regarding chrysin's ability to actually increase testosterone levels — even when used in conjunction with androgen precursor molecules — has been less than exciting. The reason for this seems to lie in the poor bio-availability (poor absorption) of chrysin. In experimental research, chrysin was shown to exert impressive increases in both total and free testosterone when it was combined with a specialized extract of pepper called piperine (known by the trade name Bioperine®). In the study, the chrysin/piperine combination was able to raise testosterone levels by 40 percent, all the while decreasing estradiol (the body's main estrogen) by close to 40 percent. The best part of all was that these results were experienced within 30 days.

As you can see, by enhancing the absorption of chrysin, one should be able to naturally elevate testosterone levels. But what is chrysin exactly, and where can you find it?

Chrysin is actually part of the flavone class of flavonoids, which are powerful antioxidants known to neutralize free radicals (free radicals are produced during oxidation and known to cause cell damage and potentially lead to a large number of major medical problems, including increased risk for stroke and heart disease). Chrysin can be found in the following:

- ❖ Passiflora coerulea
- ❖ Pelargonium crispum (geranium species)
- ❖ Pinaceae (pine trees)
- ❖ Honey

Unless you really like honey or are a die-hard vegan, it may be challenging finding a convenient natural source of chrysin. For this reason, perhaps the best source of chrysin is an all-natural health supplement. But again, synthetic nutrients tend to have low bio-availability meaning the body does not actually use very much, if any, of the nutrient, making all-natural supplements a better choice.

As mentioned before, testosterone levels are dropping from one generation to the next. Lower testosterone levels have been linked to a wide range of physical and psychological problems, making it vital for men to preserve existing levels. Inhibiting aromatase activity lowers or stops the loss of testosterone due to estrogen conversion. Although in vivo (in or on living tissue) studies are necessary, chrysin already appears to be one of the most promising tools in the fight against testosterone loss. Anyone serious about fighting andropause should consider adding chrysin to their daily diet.

Beta Sitosterol

According to the Centers for Disease Control (CDC), prostate cancer is a huge health concern for men as they grow older, and is the second leading cause of death for men in the United States. At one time, it was believed that testosterone itself may actually increase the risk for prostate cancer, and unfortunately this is still one of the predominant beliefs today.

Why is this unfortunate? Because new research shows that the *opposite* is true: the loss of testosterone *increases* the risk for prostate cancer because it leads to higher levels of "bad" estrogens like estradiol and 16-alpha-hydroxyestrone metabolites (16-OHE), and lower levels of "good" estrogens like 2-alpha-hydroxyestrone metabolites (2-OHE). Higher levels of 16-OHE are believed to lower the production of detoxifying cells that help inhibit cancer growth in the prostate, so the *loss* of testosterone actually *increases* the risk for prostate cancer.

Benign prostatic hyperplasia (BPH), or an enlarged prostate, is also thought to be caused by the loss of testosterone. Unfortunately, testosterone levels start dropping in men starting in the mid-20's primarily due to the aromatase enzyme, which we've just discussed.

A substance called *Beta sitosterol* has emerged as a potent weapon in both the fight against prostate enlargement and prostate cancer. Literally found in every single vegetable you eat, beta sitosterol is also known as plant alcohol, or a phytosterol.

Beta Sitosterol's Effect on BPH.

In one of the largest and most comprehensive studies on beta sitosterol and BPH, 200 males participated in a double blind study for one year. Not only did the study conclude that beta sitosterol effectively helped treat and alleviate symptoms of BPH, it also helped improve the overall health of the urinary tract itself.

In a shorter but more compelling 6-week study conducted at the University of Brussels, the effectiveness of beta sitosterol in treating BPH and improving urinary tract health was even more pronounced. The study concluded beta sitosterol effectively improved every characteristic of BPH on the International Prostate Symptom Score, including:

- ❖ Improved urinary flow rates
- ❖ Improved residual urinary volume
- ❖ Reduced prostate size
- ❖ Improved overall quality of Life

Although more research is needed to understand precisely how it improves urinary tract health and symptoms related to BPH, the conclusions in this study were accepted by over 88% of researchers who reviewed it. Beta sitosterol definitely helps reduce problems with an enlarged prostate but can it also help with prostate cancer?

Beta Sitosterol and Prostate Cancer

Research shows that beta sitosterol has a pronounced affect on prostate cancer cell growth. In one study involving mice that were injected with human prostate cancer cells and then given either a 2 percent solution of beta sitosterol or a 2 percent cholesterol solution, the results were positively amazing. For the mice given the 2 percent beta sitosterol solution, the growth of prostate cancer cells was inhibited by over 70 percent, versus just 18 percent with the cholesterol solution. While this may have been an *in vitro* study (meaning it was conducted in a lab setting outside of the body) involving only mice, the inhibition of prostate cancer cell growth was both significant and encouraging.

Another study, this time involving humans, was even more encouraging. It studied the effectiveness of beta sitosterol on an androgen-dependent form of prostate cancer called LNCaP. The results were certainly encouraging:

- ❖ 24 percent decrease in cancer cell growth
- ❖ 400 percent increase in apoptosis (programmed cancer cell death)
- ❖ 50 percent increase in ceramide production

Ceramides are important in the fight against cancer because they induce *apoptosis*, however researchers were unable to isolate how beta sitosterol increased their levels by such a significant amount. More studies are already under way to find out.

While men face progressively lower testosterone levels from the mid-twenties onward, which increases the risk for BPH and prostate cancer, beta sitosterol can definitely help turn the tide and put the odds back in your favor. In study after study, beta sitosterol has proved to be one of the biggest weapons in our fight against BPH and prostate cancer. Despite beta sitosterol being found in every single vegetable we eat, most people do not get enough of it (only around 200-400mg) in their daily diet. This is partly due to the fact that no one food is known to have exceptionally high levels of beta sitosterol, making supplements the best way to help protect your overall prostate health.

Indoles—Indole-3 Carbinol

Although some very compelling research suggests that

environmental toxins may cause lower testosterone levels, the fact remains that men face a natural decline of this special sex hormone simply due to aging and normal bodily processes. The good news is that it is possible to naturally combat the symptoms of testosterone loss with something known as *indole-3 carbinol*, or as it is commonly referred, I3C.

I3C is a cruciferous plant compound found in foods like broccoli and cauliflower. I3C holds great promise in helping to reduce symptoms of andropause and greatly lower the risk of prostate cancer because studies have shown that it effectively downgrades estrogen. For men, bad estrogens like 16-OHE are suspected to increase the risk for prostate cancer because they suppress other cancer-inhibiting cells in the body.

The so-called *bad* estrogens have actually been shown to be responsible for the proliferation or spreading of all known prostate cancers, especially the most aggressive ones. Studies conclude that I3C actually suppresses these bad estrogens, thus preventing them from triggering the growth and proliferation of some forms of prostate cancer.

Not only does I3C help prevent prostate cancer, research also shows that it can actually induce apoptosis (programmed cell death, a good thing when talking about cancer) in prostate cancer cells and potentially be effective in treating existing conditions. A study conducted at the Wayne State University School of Medicine revealed that I3C increases the expression of special enzymes known for their ability to detoxify and inhibit carcinogens. By encouraging the expression of these enzymes, I3C helped inhibit prostate cancer cell growth. As a result, researchers concluded I3C to be effective in both the prevention and treatment of prostate cancer.

More research is needed to fully take advantage of I3C in the fight against prostate cancer, and to understand precisely how it affects overall health, as well. But for men facing declining testosterone levels and increased problems due to andropause, I3C can be seen as a powerful ally in the fight to maintain a cancer-free prostate. I3C also helps men facing andropause symptoms because it helps promote male health in three important ways, including:

- ❖ downgrading estrogen and helping to maintain healthier estrogen to testosterone levels
- ❖ preventing the spread and/or proliferation of prostate cancer by limiting bad androgen activity
- ❖ increasing activity of detoxifying enzymes thought to inhibit cancer cell growth

Certain environmental factors may indeed be lowering testosterone levels, but our own bodies may be the most significant threat to "estrogen dominance," leading to andropause and increased risk of prostate cancer. By providing the body with healthy natural compounds like I3C that help restore a healthy hormone balance and inhibit cancer cell growth, you can safely reduce the symptoms and problems caused by testosterone loss while helping promote healthy prostate function.

Although you can find I3C in foods like broccoli, Brussels sprouts and cauliflower, modern food processing and even cooking can deplete nutritional value and rob you of their potential benefits. Therefore, it is best to include all natural I3C supplements in your daily diet to receive the prostate-healthy benefits of this amazing compound.

Stinging Nettle Root

Testosterone may be vital to men's overall physical and mental health, but it also has two powerful enemies: the aromatase enzyme, which converts testosterone into estrogen; and SHBG, which binds to testosterone and renders it useless. Luckily, there is a substance available that has been shown to be effective in countering these testosterone enemies – *stinging nettle root.*

Stinging nettle root is a wild herb found in many parts of the world, including the United States, and known to provide a number of medicinal benefits, including anti-inflammatory and anti-viral properties, and as a pain reliever. The "roots" of stinging nettle go back far indeed, and can be traced to ancient Greece when it was used to treat a number of conditions, including chronic coughs, arthritis, tuberculosis and hair loss.

One study concluded that the leaves of the stinging nettle have anti-inflammatory properties that help alleviate symptoms related to allergies. Stinging nettle leaves have also been used to "sting" the skin at the joints to relieve arthritis pain, and there is research to support them being effective for this use. But for men looking to maintain existing testosterone levels, it is the root of the stinging nettle that appears most valuable.

The Root of the Matter

Stinging nettle root has emerged as a valuable ally in the fight to maintain testosterone levels because it contains active compounds that literally compete for binding sites on SHBG, thereby freeing up more bio-available testosterone. This actually provides a double benefit for men, because not only does SHBG reduce free testosterone levels, it also binds to prostate tissue, making it more susceptible to cancer cell growth. Other studies have confirmed that stinging nettle root not only helps protect prostate cells against cancer, it literally inhibits prostate cancer cell growth.

An enlarged prostate (also known as benign prostatic hyperplasia, or BPH) is another big problem that affects millions of men as they grow older. Two enzymes, 5-alpha-reductase and aromatase, are thought to be responsible for an enlarged prostate because both reduce the ratio of testosterone to estrogen as men age. 5-alpha-reductase also elevates levels of DHT, commonly referred to as the "bad" male hormone. Stinging nettle root reduces the activity of these two enzymes, making it a powerful addition in the fight against andropause and an enlarged prostate. Even more encouraging are studies showing stinging nettle not only helps prevent enlargement of the prostate, it also helps in treating mild forms of BPH.

More research is required to determine precisely how stinging nettle root affects 5-alpha-reductase and aromatase activity, as well as impacting overall prostate size. However, the research clearly indicates that the active compounds in stinging nettle root do bind to SHBG and thus help increase free testosterone levels and protect the prostate against cancer cell *growth*.

But how do you get your hands on it, and is it safe to use? Wild stinging nettle grows throughout much of the U.S., Canada, and Europe. One should, however, err on the side of caution when picking nettle as the leaves can literally sting the skin (hence, its name), causing a rash. Although the rash can sometimes be uncomfortable and cause the affected area to feel numb, it is considered relatively harmless.

If your goal is to enhance your free testosterone levels and help protect against an enlarged prostate and cancer cell growth, all-natural stinging nettle root supplements are the best way to go.

Epimedium

Not only is testosterone decline a major problem for most men, recent research indicates that men are losing it at a faster rate than previous generations. To prevent a declining libido, increased problems with erectile dysfunction and all of the other physical and psychological issues caused by testosterone loss, men need to find ways to naturally enhance and protect existing levels of this vital sex hormone.

Epimedium, also known as Horny Goat Weed, is an herb that has been used in traditional Chinese medicine for centuries to help enhance energy levels, alleviate arthritis pain, treat and/or alleviate certain forms of cancer and enhance sexual performance by boosting energy levels. Although used for centuries in China and other regions throughout Asia, epimedium is relatively new to Western science, so there are relatively few American or European studies on the herb or its potential health benefits, though many are currently under way.

Epimedium has been researched extensively in Asia, especially China, and it is a very rich source of flavonoids. Flavonoids are powerful antioxidants known to neutralize free radicals which have been linked to a number of health problems, including premature aging (andropause) and an increased risk of cancer. The high flavonoid content of epimedium may help explain why the herb has been used in traditional Chinese medicine to help treat cancer. However, for men combating testosterone loss, studies also show that the flavonoids in epimedium also inhibit excess estrogen. Although this particular study was looking into how epimedium inhibits breast cancer, you are now well aware that lower estrogen levels create a more favorable hormone balance in men.

Although flavonoids may inhibit estrogen and create a more favorable testosterone-to-estrogen ratio, the kidney may actually be the key when it comes to enhancing sexual performance with epimedium. For over 1,000 years, the Chinese have been using epimedium to boost kidney "energy" levels in order to enhance sexual performance, and recent research supports this practice. In one study conducted in China on subjects suffering from chronic kidney failure, epimedium improved both overall kidney and sexual health in a number of ways, including higher sperm count, improved erectile function, improved immune system performance and enhanced sexual arousal.

Although the study was unable to identify precisely how epimedium improved kidney health and sexual desire, the traditional Chinese use of epimedium to enhance sexual performance by boosting kidney "energy" appears to be 100% accurate. New studies are under way to find out precisely how this happens.

Just as poor kidney health can lower sexual performance and arousal, the same is also true of cancer, which can cause symptoms like pain when having intercourse, lower libido and difficulty in maintaining arousal. Epimedium has traditionally been used in Chinese medicine to treat cancer symptoms. Clinical studies show that the phytonutrient *icariin* is abundant in epimedium and may be the source of the cancer-fighting properties described in traditional Chinese medicine. One *in vitro* study showed that icariin reduced the ability of cancer cells to invade healthy tissue. Another promising study showed icariin helped induce apoptosis (programmed cell death) of cancer cells.

Researchers may not know precisely how powerful epimedium may really become in the fight against cancer, but current research confirms that it does have cancer-inhibiting properties and may very well help treat it, and thus help elevate sexual interest, arousal, and pleasure.

More scientific research needs to be conducted, but according to current studies on the potent herb, epimedium does help stimulate sexual arousal, improve kidney health, and inhibit cancer cell growth. In traditional Chinese medicine, epimedium is used in powder form (5 grams, or 1 tsp) three times per day after simmering with water for about ten minutes. If not prepared properly, however, the drink can cause irritability, fever, and aggressive behavior. This is why it is best to consume epimedium in a natural supplement form.

Lycopene

As you are now well aware, in andropause, not only do testosterone levels drop, they actually become converted into estrogen. This excess estrogen (as well as its metabolites) greatly diminishes prostate health and increases the risk of prostate cancer. As testosterone levels drop and estrogen levels increase, so do bad estrogen metabolites like 16-OHE. The lowered testosterone and increased concentration of

16-OHE is believed to lower the number of cells that naturally inhibit cancer cell growth in the prostate, thus increasing the risk of prostate cancer. The loss of testosterone has also been linked with increased risk for BPH.

Since 16-OHE and other forms of estrogen ultimately lower testosterone levels and increase the risk of poor prostate health, it is comforting to know that there are powerful natural wonders from the plant kingdom that can help us combat andropause and protect ourselves against BPH and prostate cancer. Recent research indicates that *lycopene*, abundant in tomatoes, may be such a nutrient.

Lycopene is actually a carotenoid, a powerful class of antioxidants that can neutralize free radical damage. Free radicals have been linked to premature aging and almost all forms of cancer, including prostate and colon. In addition to fighting off free radicals, lycopene can also help remove toxins from the body.

Lycopene and Prostate Cancer

The common tomato has long been rumored to have medicinal benefits, but only recently have scientists isolated pure lycopene as a potential cancer-fighting agent. In a recent study conducted by researchers at the Harvard Medical School, participants consuming two to four servings daily over a 6-year period of tomato products reduced the risk for prostate cancer by 35%. Even frequent (less than daily) consumption of tomato products significantly reduced prostate cancer risks.

Lycopene and Enlarged Prostate

An enlarged prostate can cause frequent urinating and a number of other discomforting problems that can lead to even bigger medical issues down the road, even prostate cancer itself. Testosterone loss may lead to problems with BPH, but researchers have learned that lycopene can literally stop BPH in its tracks. In one study using 40 patients with BPH, half were given just 15 mg/day of lycopene while the other half received a placebo. While the prostate grew larger for the placebo group, those receiving lycopene did not have further enlargement and also showed reduced symptoms of BPH, according to the International Prostate Symptom Score. Imagine, if simply by eating tomatoes and thereby getting your daily dose of lycopene, you could actually help halt prostate enlargement while reducing your risk of prostate cancer.

But not so fast, it isn't *quite* that simple. It turns out that lycopene is activated only when tomatoes are cooked, which is why tomato sauce seems to be a much better way to get your lycopene fix than is eating a raw tomato. Researchers are not exactly certain how lycopene promotes prostate health, but study after study concludes that it does indeed deliver these preventative benefits. Some speculate those health benefits are due to lycopene being a carotenoid, and thus a powerful antioxidant that can remove toxins and inhibit cancer cell growth. Others believe lycopene affects the testosterone-to-estrogen ratio and somehow slows or even reverses the effects of andropause, thus promoting overall prostate health.

Whatever the exact mechanism, lycopene appears to be very good for the prostate. Prostate cancer is the second leading cause of death for men in the United States and a very real health concern for millions of aging men. Lycopene has proven effective in preventing BPH from progressing further and in reducing the risk of prostate cancer, but some may have a hard time incorporating tomato-based foods in their daily diet. For anyone with acid reflux or digestive problems, tomatoes are acidic and can aggravate symptoms. All-natural lycopene supplements are a great way to help protect your prostate and perhaps the most convenient way to include this vital carotenoid in your daily diet.

Zinc (for the Dink)

Like vitamin C and other common nutrients, somewhere in the back of our minds we all know that *zinc* is good for us and should be included in our daily diet, but few of us really understand exactly why. For any man worried about or suffering from symptoms related to testosterone loss and andropause, maintaining adequate zinc levels becomes paramount. Recent research indicates that male testosterone levels can drop due to a zinc deficiency. In one study on the effects of zinc deficiency and supplementation, one group of healthy males were purposely given a diet low in zinc. After six months, their testosterone levels had dropped by nearly 75%. In the other group, older men (aged 55-70) already suffering from low testosterone levels and a minor zinc deficiency were given zinc supplements, and after six months, their serum testosterone levels had nearly doubled.

While these findings may seem incredible or hard to believe, the research was actually building upon a previous study which found men with a zinc deficiency also suffered from low testosterone levels and a low sperm count. These findings are less surprising when one understands that zinc is actually excreted in the prostate and is also released in sperm during ejaculation. In fact, a study conducted at the world famous Karolinka Institute in Stockholm, Sweden found that men with high sperm counts also had higher levels of zinc in their sperm, so the evidence points to a very strong relationship between zinc, sperm, and higher testosterone levels.

Although scientists don't yet know precisely how zinc affects testosterone levels, it seems that zinc plays a central roll in helping to regulate testosterone metabolism. Further research is under way to confirm this theory. However, while the link between zinc and testosterone levels has been confirmed by clinical studies, there seems to be a big mystery: millions of men around the world take supplements with zinc in them and yet still suffer from low or declining testosterone levels. How is this possible? The answer is bio-availability, the make-it-or-break-it factor for nearly every supplement we've discussed.

Bio-Availability
Simply put, bio-availability refers to the ability of the body to absorb and actually use a particular nutrient, including zinc. Low bio-availability means the body absorbs very little of a given nutrient while high bio-availability is just the opposite. The problem with many supplements is that they incorporate various forms of zinc with very low bio-availability, like zinc oxide or zinc sulfate. Zinc bio-availability can also be reduced by other minerals, such as calcium. Gluconate, citrate and amino acid-bound zinc supplements (Aminomin™) have a higher bio-availability and are easier for the body to absorb, so shop for supplements made with these forms of the mineral for best results.

The RDA for zinc is 15 mg for men, but consider your age and activity level when reading the labels on this and all other supplements. As the body ages it becomes more difficult to absorb nutrients like zinc, so a supplement with only 15 mg may not be adequate to maintain or boost testosterone levels. Plus, the body loses zinc as it sweats, so athletes and men with very active lifestyles may also require higher levels of zinc in their supplements to avoid becoming depleted.

Natural sources of zinc include red meat, wheat germ, oysters, and brewer's yeast. Even if you think your diet is rich in zinc, think again. Modern food processing and even cooking can rob foods of their nutrients, including zinc. Surprisingly, even athletes who are notorious for being careful about their dietary intake may suffer from zinc depletion or deficiency. A major laboratory in California tested more than 200,000 serious athletes in this regard, and a shocking 70% were either zinc depleted or deficient.

For any man serious about maintaining or boosting existing testosterone levels and avoiding the many medical problems associated with lower levels of this vital sex hormone, good old-fashioned zinc may be the answer you have been looking for.

13

The Return of Fred

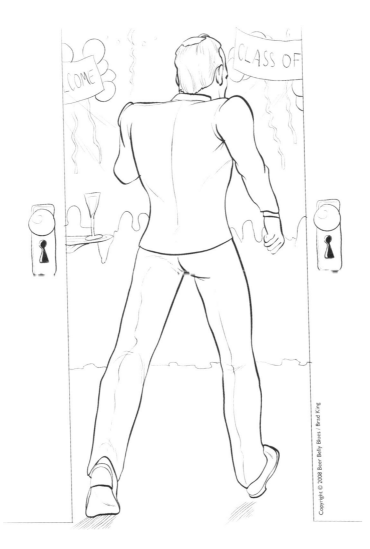

My name is Fred. And I'm a happy man.

I reintroduce myself here because I bear little resemblance to the fellow you met in these pages some three months ago, on the day I received that fateful invitation to my 25-year high school reunion. Short of a military induction notice, I can't imagine a more terrifying envelope to open, because at the time I was wallowing around in what I realized was the muck that resides at the bottom of the barrel. I was fat. I was going bald. I was negotiating a divorce. I was lonely and miserable. Okay, I was pathetic. And I was kidding myself every time I tried pass it all off as no big deal, as simply the sad reality of reaching middle age.

Life sucks, then you die. Or so I'd heard.

But this reunion was a big deal. In fact, it was my only deal. I could have just said no, thrown that invitation away and got on with my life, and I shudder to think how close I came to making that decision. Instead I took a long, hard, painful look in the mirror and had a little chat with that guy staring back at me, who was a bit of a mess. Much of my situation was of my own making, especially where my recently departed wife was concerned. Some of it, I suspected, was the product of time itself, and therefore beyond my complete control. Or so I thought.

But there was no getting around the truth: what happened next was completely within my control. Because I had 12 weeks to reinvent myself. To lose my beer belly. To get back into shape and become at least a shadow of my former elite-athlete self. To get healthy again, to feel better in general. And perhaps most importantly, to recapture some measure of self-respect and hope.

And maybe, just maybe, make my ex-wife jealous at the

reunion because some of the girls who hadn't seen me in years were going to be paying attention, just like in the old days. At least, that was my game plan.

And so it began. I went to a naturopathic physician who explained that there was more going on here than too many chips and not enough sweat. That my biochemistry had shifted with age – andropause, she called it – which, in combination with a less than healthy lifestyle (this was the too many chips and not enough sweat part), had conspired to encourage my body to decrease its production of natural testosterone. She went on to explain how a man's level of testosterone dictates many facets of his existence – his tendency to gain weight, his level of strength, hair loss, even his sexual drive and the ability to perform in the sack (which was the least of my problems at the time, but something I was certainly planning to pay attention to in the future). All of this rang true for me, and I knew that if there was a way I could turn this testosterone thing around, to somehow discover the path toward increasing my levels of natural testosterone while decreasing so-called "bad" hormones that were taking me in the wrong direction, both physically and emotionally, that I would be more than willing to make the lifestyle changes required to make it happen and make it last.

Famous last words, I know. Nobody who has ever started a diet did so with the intention of failing. No, that intention usually took about three days to manifest. But this time I was serious. There would be only one 25th year high school reunion. No second chances. Just like life itself.

And so I did it. I joined a fitness club. Put myself into the hands of a knowledgeable personal trainer who, in a gym full of poseurs doing things pretty much all wrong, showed me the right way to workout, how to lift weights and how to incorporate proper aerobic exercise into my routine (or as she called it, "high impact-short duration interval training), all of it designed to kick-start my body into a rapid weight-loss mode while jacking my level of natural testosterone in the process. With the help of my new naturopath, I completely overhauled my eating patterns, not only in terms of what I ate, but when I ate, and how often, in combination with a regimen of natural supplements (in fact, the ones you just read about). In other words, I gave my body everything it needed to make the changes required – to shed fat, to increase testosterone, even to fight disease.

I won't say it was easy, but I'll stand on the highest mountain and scream that it was all worth it. Because it worked. I lost nearly 30 pounds in 12 weeks. I rediscovered muscles I'd forgotten I'd had, and my strength returned to a level I hadn't seen since shortly after high school. Best of all, I felt great, not only because of how I looked in the mirror, but from an unexpected surge of energy and ambition. Heck, even my hair looked better.

And, I might add, I finally got back into my old letterman jacket, which had aged just as poorly as me. But it fit again. I had done it.

All in just 12 weeks. All in time for the dreaded high school reunion. Which I no longer dreaded. I couldn't wait to see the expression on my ex-wife's face when she saw me in my new clothes, with my new body and a rejuvenated sense of self-confidence. Not that I wanted her back – no, she'd moved on, and it was all for the best, since I still had relationship issues to work on. But now I had hope. And if I could make her notice, even for just a moment, I could infuse that hope with a bit more confidence, which I knew I'd need.

Here's how it all went down.

No one noticed that I'd lost weight. At first this bothered me, but when I thought about it, it made perfect sense. I hadn't seen most of my classmates in years, which means they had no idea how out of shape I'd allowed myself to become. In fact, if I hadn't lost the weight I'm pretty sure the place would have been buzzing about how I looked, and not in a good way. But those few that I had crossed paths with in recent years did notice, saying I looked great and that I'd dropped a few since back when. But for the most part, my weight was not the issue. What was the issue was that I hadn't changed all that much in the last 25 years. Or so I was told, over and over again. It felt great, but there was one opinion that mattered more than the others.

My wife – okay, ex-wife... some habits are hard to let go of, especially when you're writing an alimony check every month – arrived late, par for the course. On her arm was the new boyfriend, who as predicted looked a few years younger than the rest of us and, I have to admit, had that air of money and success that makes a guy eminently unlikable at first glance. It was a chilly introduction, but a little later the guy came over to me at the bar and said he'd heard I was the school jock, and that I still looked the part. Suddenly Mr. Richer And Younger Than Me seemed like a pretty nice guy – not that I was planning any sleepovers here – one with impeccable judgment and a keen eye for talent. He'd landed my ex, after all.

Just when I thought the entire evening would pass without my pound of flesh, my ex approached and asked me to dance with her. As we silently danced to what was once one of our favorite old songs – this being the reason for the invite, I think – she said the most amazing thing.

"I want you to know something," she said, her eyes a bit more moist that I'd seen them in years. "I'm happy. Ron's a great

guy."

"Young, too," I added.

"Don't go there, Fred. Please."

"No, really," I responded. "I never thought I'd say this, but he seems like a decent guy." I paused, then added, "I'm happy for you. Really."

Amazing what a little testosterone does for one's soul.

"Thank you." She looked away. Then it happened. "I want you to know that I'm proud of you," she said. "I mean, how you look tonight, how you're carrying yourself. Whatever you're doing, you should bottle it, because it works."

"Thirty pounds," I declared.

"It's not just that. I mean, it's the old you, Fred. The way you just are. Your smile is back. The old confidence. I haven't seen you like this in years."

She paused, the unspoken heavy between us. Then she added, "I thought that guy was gone."

Now the moisture in the eyes was mine. "Thank you," was all that I could squeak out. It wasn't the jealous pang I'd hoped for. No, this was better. I'd earned her respect. Something I hadn't been worthy of in years.

The music ended and she squeezed my hand. "See you around," she said, only with a wink that took all the venom out of it.

"Be happy," I whispered as she walked away. She stopped and looked back.

"You, too." Then she flicked her eyes toward a group of women, who I couldn't help but notice had been watching our every move. The quarterback and the homecoming queen, having a last dance together.

It was then that I realized the best part of it all was that we'd danced with absolutely no sciatic pain in my legs whatsoever. So much for the broken heart.

And now for the real best part. One of those women is now my girlfriend. We finished the reunion in a tight huddle over coffee, the last two to leave, confessing that we hadn't connected in high school because we ran in different crowds. She was a late bloomer, and said she was surprised that I even remembered her. But now, 25 years later, she was the most attractive woman in the room, a runner, a dancer, a mother, a dreamer and a self-employed consultant who didn't care how much or how little money I made. We've been seeing each other ever since. One late bloomer with another, looking forward to a future free from the worries of middle age. Two people who understood that life's too short for worry.

And, we are making love like rabbits.

They say that age is just a number, but I know better. Age can and should be a sum in excess of its parts, if and only if you know what the parts are and how to manage them. If you don't pay attention to those parts – testosterone especially – they will go their own way and send you spiraling to a slow decent, robbing you of the essence of life itself, depleting your health, strength, beauty, energy and hope.

Take it from this late bloomer – it doesn't have to go down that way. If you are experiencing any of the symptoms of low testosterone, take the information within these pages to heart and apply it.

Don't just sit there... Actually do something about it.

Too many of us do the "man thing" and put important things off for that perfect day, the old, "I'll get around to it as soon as I get a second" mantra. Only that perfect day never seems to come and that second turns into a lifetime. What could be more important than the rest of your life? Think about it.

Hey, if it can happen to me, it can happen to you, too.

And it definitely did happen to me. Quicker than you think. No more Beer Belly Blues, no more sad-sack Fred. The future looks bright, and thanks to what I now know about the information in this book, I plan on sucking up every moment of it.

I wish you happy sucking, as well.

APPENDIX I

Testing One, Two, Three

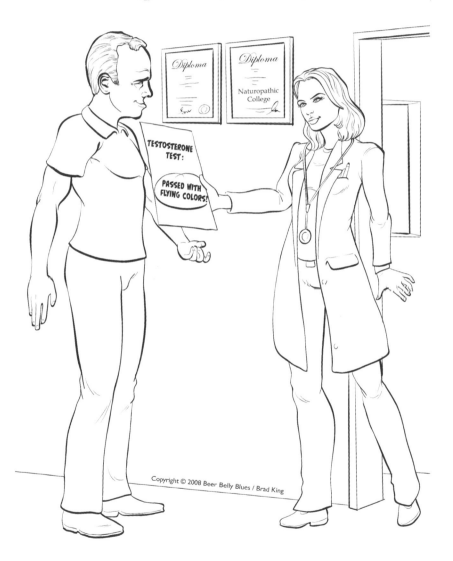

APPENDIX I
Testing One, Two, Three

Whether we're talking about sex drive or overall prostate health, nothing is more important for men then overall testosterone levels. Whether due to internal body processes or external environmental factors, the loss of testosterone is troubling for men concerned about their health.

As a brief recap: lower testosterone levels have been scientifically linked to a number of moderate to severe issues, including:

❖   Muscle Loss
❖   Weight gain (increase in body fat)
❖   Bone density loss (osteoporosis)
❖   Hair loss
❖   Insomnia and/or disruptions in normal sleep patterns
❖   Loss of interest in sex
❖   Depression
❖   Erectile dysfunction (difficulty achieving and/or maintaining an erection)
❖   Difficulty with concentration/memory
❖   Loss of energy
❖   Increased risk for cardiovascular disease

Without question, the loss of testosterone can have very serious consequences for a man's physical, mental, and sexual health. The good news is you are now well-armed in various tactics of combating testosterone loss through effective lifestyle, diet, exercise and supplementation protocols. Each of the strategies discussed in this book, especially when combined, can help enhance existing testosterone levels, reduce the level of natural age-related loss, and even help alleviate symptoms.

The first step in the process is to find out if you are presently experiencing less than adequate levels of testosterone. In order to know for sure (besides the many obvious signs listed throughout this book), you'll need to have your testosterone levels checked.

Who should consider having testosterone levels tested?

Any man over age 35, or any man experiencing one or more of the symptoms listed above should have their testosterone tested on a regular basis.

Testing Options - Blood vs. Salivary

In a laboratory setting, blood tests are most common and usually involve a small sample taken from the arm in the early morning when testosterone levels are highest. However, do-it-yourself at home tests are also available and measure levels in the saliva (salivary tests). For anyone experiencing symptoms of testosterone loss, the blood test is definitely recommended. But for anyone just looking to monitor testosterone levels as they age, the saliva tests can help identify emerging problems. Users simply have to collect saliva at specified times during the day and then mail the sample to the lab or the company providing the test. Results usually take two to three weeks.

What if testosterone replacement is required?

In some cases of low testosterone, a qualified health professional may recommend a regimen of testosterone therapy using prescription-only products. In this case it is always best to discuss bio-identical testosterone replacement with your physician.

Bio-identical testosterone is best taken as a topically-applied cream purchased from a compounding pharmacy. These compounded testosterone creams are able to supply the same testosterone produced in your body at precise amounts that are easily absorbed into the bloodstream. This is also the best way to approximate the way testosterone is *naturally* produced – or at least should be – by the body each day. Compounded testosterone creams are much less expensive than brand-name testosterone creams or gels. (NOTE: in rare instances as determined by your physician, testosterone injections are the next best choice versus topically-applied creams.)

It is always wise to avoid oral ingestion of testosterone in the form of pills, as oral testosterone is quickly degraded by liver enzymes, which more often than not leads to unhealthy variations in blood levels of testosterone and possible liver problems.

Recommended Male Panel Tests

Blood and salivary tests are the two basic options for testosterone testing, but there are several other specific male panel tests to consider, including:

❖   Free Testosterone (Total Testosterone)
❖   Estradiol
❖   Pregnenolone
❖   DHEA Sulfate
❖   Lipid Profile
❖   TSH (Thyroid Stimulating Hormone)
❖   PSA (Total and Free)
❖   CRP (C-Reactive Protein)

The following is a brief overview of each test.

Free Testosterone (Total Testosterone)

It is extremely important to understand that testosterone exists in two primary forms in the body: *free* and *bound*. Free testosterone refers to the amount of the sex hormone actually available to the body for use — that is, it is not bound. Testosterone can be bound by either Albumin (a serum protein) or Sex Hormone Binding Globulin (SHBG). Albumin is considered a rather weak binding agent that the body can easily break and therefore it uses most testosterone that is bound to it. SHBG, on the other hand, forms a strong bond that is very difficult for the body to break so any testosterone bound to it is not considered to be free or usable by the body.

Unfortunately, many testosterone tests measure the total testosterone present in the blood, which includes both free and bound versions. This does not present a clear picture of how much testosterone is actually available to the body and is therefore not considered to be a comprehensive measure of existing levels. An *equilibrium dialysis* test is considered superior to a total test because it measures free testosterone *plus* a portion of the albumin-bound testosterone while excluding any hormones bound to SHBG. This is a much clearer indication of the amount of testosterone available to the body for use, but the costs of this test are greater. However, to get the clearest picture possible of "usable" testosterone, the added costs are well worth it.

So what results should you hope for with a testosterone test? That answer actually depends on a lot of factors. But remember, blood test laboratory reference ranges are age-adjusted, reflecting the anticipated reduction in testosterone that almost all men experience. So optimum levels should be near the higher end of that range.

The following are considered normal ranges for most men and women:

Men: 300-1200 ng/DL
Women: 30-95 ng/DL

Because "normal" testosterone levels depend upon age, it is important to consult with a physician to determine whether or not your particular levels are low, high, or normal.

Estradiol

Yes, estradiol is a form of estrogen (actually it is the primary estrogen from which all other estrogens are made) and is considered to be primarily a female hormone, though it is found in both men and women. For men, levels increase when testosterone is converted into estrogen via the aromatase enzyme. Elevated levels of estradiol have been associated with increased risk for prostate cancer while extremely low levels can increase the risk of bone fractures and lower bone density. Because it is so important to male health for estradiol levels not to be too high or low, testing becomes increasingly vital as men age due to the increased fluctuations of this hormone.

Pregnenolone

Although it may be difficult to locate a facility that tests pregnenolone levels, this hormone actually plays a huge role in the aging process. Pregnenolone is actually a building block vital to the production of several other important hormones, including: testosterone, DHEA, estrogen and progesterone. But just as with overall testosterone levels, the body begins producing less and less pregnenolone beginning in the early to mid-30s. For men facing andropause, pregnenolone is an important ally because it is likely to be converted into testosterone if levels are low. Pregnenolone is also useful in fighting other problems associated with aging, such as fatigue and poor memory. Studies even show it can stimulate brain cell growth.

DHEA (sulfate)

Perhaps ironically, DHEA levels are typically only tested when an excess of testosterone is suspected because it can indicate the presence of tumors in the adrenal gland. However, because testosterone is also produced in the adrenal glands, testing for DHEA is also important for anyone facing andropause or any of its symptoms. Low levels of DHEA can indicate a problem in adrenal gland function (including high cortisol) and a potential source of low testosterone levels.

TSH (Thyroid Stimulating Hormone)

The TSH test basically assesses thyroid gland function, which affects growth, development, and body metabolism. Hypothyroidism (low thyroid function is signified by the production of too much TSH, and can produce symptoms that resemble many andropause issues, including loss of energy, muscle weakness, depression, hair loss and weight gain) has also been linked with increased risk for cardiovascular disease.

Even though TSH readings are considered normal at levels up to 5.5 mU/L, research indicates that the optimal range of TSH is below 2.0 mU/L.

Lipid Profile

As the name suggests, a lipid profile does not really look at testosterone levels. Rather, it looks at total cholesterol, HDL, LDL, and triglycerides. The purpose of a lipid profile is ultimately to determine the risk for coronary artery disease. Low testosterone levels have been linked with increased risk of coronary artery disease, so a lipid profile is merely a precautionary test usually performed in conjunction with a testosterone test and will likely be recommended by your physician. A lipid profile is definitely recommended for anyone who:

- ❖ Smokes cigarettes/tobacco products
- ❖ Is over the age of 45 for men, 55 for women
- ❖ Has hypertension (blood pressure above 140/90)
- ❖ Has family history of coronary heart disease

PSA (Total and Free)

Prostate Specific Antigen, or PSA, is a protein produced naturally in the prostate gland. Elevated levels may be an indication of problems in the prostate, particularly prostate cancer. Many physicians believe that a PSA test is vital, though it is important to note that the PSA has one of the highest false-positive rates of any medical test — as high as 85%. In fact, one well-controlled study that appeared in the *New England Journal of Medicine* (1991) showed that 78% of men who scored high on the PSA (between 4—10), showed no trace of cancer when subjected to a biopsy.

The total PSA test should be used in conjunction with a digital rectal exam (DRE) and is often performed on men already suffering with prostate cancer to help verify the effectiveness of treatment. However, a total PSA can also be used on patients with prostate cancer symptoms, such as difficult, painful and/or infrequent urination, as well as back pain and pelvic pain. Most doctors will recommend a biopsy when elevated levels of PSA are indicated, though you should always ask for a second or third opinion before going this route. The total PSA is currently believed to be the best way to assess prostate health without a biopsy, and the American Cancer Association recommends an annual total PSA test for men starting at age 50.

A healthy PSA reading is below 4.0 ng/mL, with free-PSA above 25% (free-PSA is lower in people with prostate cancer).

CRP (C-Reactive Protein)

The CRP test is used to help assess overall heart health, which is a major concern for men with low testosterone levels, as the test can help determine an increased risk for coronary heart disease. Aside from this it is also a very effective measure of overall inflammation in the body (inflammation is one of the key causes of coronary heart disease).

Crohn's disease, or inflammatory bowel disease, is another problem men face as they get older. Elevated CRP levels indicate the presence of infection or inflammation, so testing for this protein can help identify potential problems with intestinal disorders as well.

Normally, levels of CRP hover below 10mg/L, but the presence of an infection or inflammation can send them above 100mg/L. making it easy to identify a potential problem.

All of the tests mentioned above are vital to men and can help identify potential health problems relating to testosterone loss in time to treat them. While not all tests look specifically at testosterone or even hormone levels, all of the Male Panel Tests mentioned here will help promote male health by identifying potential problems associated with aging, including andropause. The most important tests of all are, of course, those that test for free and total testosterone. Because testosterone is the elixir of life and health for men, and testing for it should be an integral part of health maintenance and care.

APPENDIX II

The Ultimate Way to Supplement

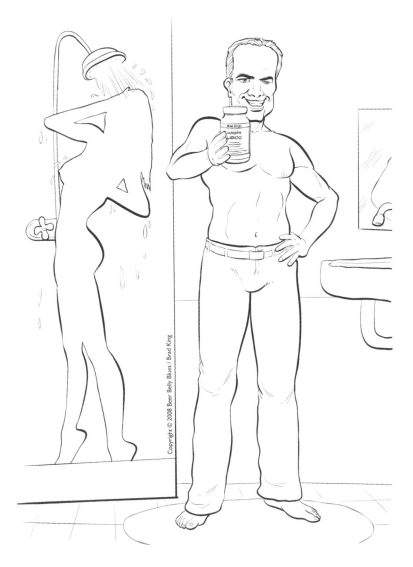

APPENDIX II
The Ultimate Way to Supplement

In chapter 12 and throughout other sections of Beer Belly Blues, there has been mention of various nutrients that offer special benefits where overall health, especially male health, is concerned. Many of these nutrients can be found in synergistic combinations within special formulas mentioned below.

What constitutes a great product?

In my many years in the health industry, I have come to realize that a nutrient formula is only as good as the quality of its starting ingredients as well as the manufacturing practices used to create it. It is therefore imperative to have all bases covered when creating a high quality nutrient formula. The criteria I have used as a product formulator over the years is as follows:

❖ First off, there has to be a real need for the specific product

❖ all ingredients within the formula need to be of the highest quality

❖ all ingredients within the formula need to be researched based and in the ratios and/or extracts found in the studies that support their efficacy

❖ all ingredients within the formula need to work in synergy

❖ each new production batch must be third party verified for quality assurance

All products in the Ultimate line meet the above criteria and are amongst the best – if not the best – products in the industry.

Note: Since I am an avid supporter of the health food industry, most of the recommended supplements in this section can be found throughout Canada at local health food retailers. If you presently reside outside of Canada, you can find these formulas on-line at **www.AwakenYourBody.com.** The reason we do not sell on-line to Canadians, is because we are committed to supporting the health food stores in which these products are carried.

All Ultimate products are distributed (exclusively through health food stores) in Canada by:
Preferred Nutrition Inc.
Order Desk: 1-888-826-9625
Fax: 1-888-773-7069
www.pno.ca

Outside Canada:
On-line only: www.AwakenYourBody.com

Following is a brief description of each Ultimate formula. Under each formula you will find a list of ingredients that are mentioned in chapter 12. This list *does not* account for all ingredients found in that formula. For more information, including all ingredients and dosages, on each formula, please visit **www.AwakenYourBody.com** and click on the products icon:

The following Ultimate Proteins are the best tasting 100% naturally sweetened and flavored whey protein isolates available today — Garanteed!

Ultimate High-Alpha Whey Protein™
The Ultimate High-Alpha Whey Protein™ is a one-of-a-kind high performance functional protein that contains the highest

levels of the bioactive peptide *alpha-lactalbumin* – nature's most perfect form of protein. The exceptionally high levels of bioactive proteins, peptides and amino acids are obtained through an exclusive low-heat, cross flow micro-filtration method that filters out all impurities and guarantees a completely bioavailable, high performance functional protein coming from 100% whey isolate (no inexpensive, less bioavailable concentrate). The result is a protein that can actually impact the body's biological systems and help lower stress hormones (cortisol), balance moods, reduce cravings, aid in deep restorative sleep (i.e. supporting optimal HGH production) and boost energy levels during the day. Ultimate High-Alpha Whey Protein™ is garanteed to contain a minimum of 33% alpha-lactalbumin.

What to expect from this product

The unique levels of bioactive proteins, peptides and amino acids within Ultimate High-Alpha Whey Protein™ play a number of significant health enhancing roles in the body, some of which include (but are not limited to):

- building, repairing and replacing body cells for faster recuperation
- building and repairing muscle, skin and bones
- reducing appearance of wrinkles
- promoting healthy hair and nails
- improving metabolism (i.e. fat loss)
- balancing immunity for greater defense against disease
- effectively reducing stress
- effectively lowering cortisol
- enhancing feel-good brain chemicals (serotonin and dopamine)
- aiding in efficient sleep

Ultimate Iso-Energy™

Ultimate Iso-Energy™ uses only the highest quality whey isolate and takes it to the next level with a gentle low-heat cross flow micro-filtration method that filters out all impurities and guarantees a completely undenatured high quality whey isolate (no inexpensive, less bioavailable concentrate). Ultimate Iso-Energy™ contains the industries highest levels of powerful immune enhancing peptides called GMPs (28%) which have been shown to be anti-microbial, anti-bacterial and anti-viral. The exceptionally high GMP levels make Ultimate Iso-Energy™ an important addition to anyones health enhancing program (especially athletes and the elderly).

What to expect from this product

The unique peptides within Ultimate Iso-Energy™ play a number of significant health enhancing rolls in the body, some of which include (but are not limited to):

- ❖ building, repairing and replacing body cells
- ❖ building and repairing muscle, skin and bones
- ❖ improving metabolism (i.e. fat loss)
- ❖ enhancing immunity and health
- ❖ providing more energy for the body
- ❖ regulating many important metabolic processes
- ❖ providing optimal intracellular hydration

The remaining products are specifically designed to offer maximum nutritional support to the body, optimize free-testosterone levels, reduce estrogens (including the harmful estrogen metabolites) and block harmful DHT levels for optimal prostate support.

For a detailed description of each product and its ingredients please visit **www.AwakenYourBody.com** and click on the products icon.

Ultimate Multi Maximum-Performance™

The Ultimate Multi Maximum-Performance™ is the most complete multi vitamin/mineral formula available today. The formula contains optimal daily levels of all essential nutrients in their most bioavailable forms. There truly is no other multi vitamin/mineral formula that can compare in quality or value.

Ultimate Male Energy™

Ultimate Male Energy™ contains a synergistic blend of the following 100% natural ingredients:

- ❖ Chrysin
- ❖ Stinging Nettle Root
- ❖ Indole-3-Carbinol
- ❖ Bioperine® (black pepper extract)

The formula helps restore healthy, youthful hormone balance by positively affecting testosterone production and helping to lower excess estrogens.

Ultimate Prostate™

Ultimate Prostate™ contains a synergistic blend of the following 100% natural ingredients:

- ❖ Beta sitosterol (non-genetically modified)
- ❖ Stinging nettle root
- ❖ Lycopene
- ❖ Indole-3-Carbinol
- ❖ Zinc (Aminomin™)
- ❖ Bioperine® (black pepper extract)

The formula helps restore healthy prostate function and reduce urinary frequency (BPH) by blocking harmful DHT levels as well as reducing harmful estrogens (and their metabolites).

Ultimate Libido™

Ultimate Libido™ contains a synergistic blend of the following 100% natural ingredients:

- ❖ Tongkat Ali (100:1 extract from Malaysia)
- ❖ Epimedium
- ❖ Zinc (Aminomin™)
- ❖ Bioperine® (black pepper extract)

The formula helps enhance all facets of libido by naturally working to elevate free-testosterone levels.

Ultimate Maca™

Ultimate Maca™ contains 100% certified organic Peruvian Maca that has had its fiber and starch removed through a unique gelatinization process to maximize absorption and bioavailability.

For more information please visit
www.AwakenYourBody.com

Bibliography

All references in alphabetical order.

Part 1
Singing the Beer Belly Blues

Chapter 1
The Birth of the Beer Belly

Badr FM, et al. Suppression of testosterone production by ethyl alcohol. Possible mode of action. Steroids. 1977 Nov;30(5):647-55.

Campbell WW, et al. Effects of an omnivorous diet compared with a lactoovovegetarian diet on resistance-training-induced changes in body composition and skeletal muscle in older men. Am J Clin Nutr. 1999 Dec;70(6):1032-9.

Feldman HA, et al. Age trends in the level of serum testosterone and other hormones in middle-aged men: longitudinal results from the Massachusetts male aging study. J Clin Endocrinol Metab. 2002 Feb;87(2):589-98.

Hannak D, et al. Acetate formation after short-term ethanol administration in man. Biol Chem Hoppe Seyler 1985; 366:749–53.

Hsieh C., et al.; "Predictors of Sex Hormone Levels among the Elderly: A Study in Greece." J. Clin Epid 51, no. 10 (October 1998):837–841.

Hsieh, C., P. Björntorp. "The Interactions between Hypothalamic-Pituitary-Adrenal Axis Activity, Testosterone, Insulin-like Growth Factor I and Abdominal Obesity with Metabolism and Blood Pressure in Men." Int J Obes Relat Metab Disord 22, no. 12 (1998): 1184-1196.

Kalyani RR, Dobs AS. Androgen deficiency, diabetes, and the metabolic syndrome in men. Curr Opin Endocrinol Diabetes Obes. 2007 Jun;14(3):226-34.

King BJ, Schmidt MA. Bio-Age: 10 Steps to a Younger You. CDG Books Canada. 2001.

Lemon PW. Effects of exercise on dietary protein requirements. Int J Sport Nutr. 1998 Dec;8(4):426-47

Lundquist F, et al. Ethanol metabolism and production of free acetate in the human liver. J Clin Invest 1962;41:955–61.

Lundquist F. Production and utilization of free acetate in man. Nature 1962;193:579–80.

Mehmet O, Roizen M. You: An Owners Manual. Harper Collins Publishers, New York, NY 2005.

Morley JE. Andropause, testosterone therapy, and quality of life in aging men. Cleve Clin J Med. 2000 Dec;67(12):880-2.

Ravaglia G, et al. Determinants of functional status in healthy Italian nonagenarians and centenarians: a comprehensive functional assessment by the instruments of geriatric practice. J Am Geriatr Soc. 1997 Oct;45(10):1196-202.

Rosmond, R., and P. Björntorp. "Endocrine and Metabolic Aberrations in Men with Abdominal Obesity in Relation to Anxio-depressive Infirmity." Metabolism 47, no. 10 (1998):1187-1193.

Siler, S.Q., et al. De novo lipogenesis, lipid kinetics, and whole-body lipid balances in humans after acute alcohol consumption. Amer J. Clin Nut, 70, 928-936, 1999.

Svartberg J, et al. Waist circumference and testosterone levels in community dwelling men. The Tromsø study. Eur J Epidemiol, 19: 657-663, 2004

Tchernof, A., et al. "Relationships Between Endogenous Steroid Hormone, Sex Hormone-Binding Globulin and Lipoprotein Levels in Men: Contribution of Visceral Obesity, Insulin Levels and Other Metabolic Variables." Atherosclerosis 133, no. 2 (September 1997):235-244.

Valimaki, M.J., et al. Sex hormones and adrenocortical steroids in men acutely intoxicated with ethanol. Alcohol, 1, 89-93, 1984.

Volpi E, et al. Exogenous amino acids stimulate net muscle protein synthesis in the elderly. J Clin Invest. 1998 May 1;101(9):2000-7.

Chapter 2
Oh, My Aching Back...and Knees... and Shoulders...

Brennan FM, et al. Role of pro-inflammatory cytokines in rheumatoid arthritis. Springer Semin Immunopathol. 1998;20(1-2):133-47.

Crofford LJ. COX-1 and COX-2 tissue expression: implications and predictions. J Rheumatol 1997; 24 (suppl 49):15-19.

David MJ. Effect of non-steroidal anti-inflammatory drugs (NSAIDS) on glycosyltransferase activity from human osteoarthritic cartilage. Br J Rheumatol. 1992;31 Suppl 1:13-7.

Dingle JT. The effect of NSAIDs on human articular cartilage glycosaminoglycan synthesis. Eur J Rheum Inflam 1996;16:47-52.

Griffin MR. Pain Relief: How NSAIDs Work. WebMD feature article.

Hansen JM, de Muckadell OB. Selective COX-2 inhibitors--side effects in relation to non-specific non-steroidal anti-inflammatory drugs. Ugeskr Laeger. 2004 Dec 6;166(50):4581-4.

James WH. Further evidence that low androgen values are a cause of rheumatoid arthritis: the response of rheumatoid arthritis to seriously stressful life events. Ann Rheum Dis. 1997 Sep;56(9):566

King BJ. Conquer Inflammation. Transforming Health Inc. 2006.

Klegeris A, McGeer PL. Cyclooxygenase and 5-lipoxygenase inhibitors protect against mononuclear phagocyte neurotoxicity. Neurobiol Aging. 2002 Sep-Oct;23(5):787-94.

Lanas A. Gastrointestinal and cardiovascular side effects associated with COX-2 selective inhibitors. Med Clin (Barc). 2002 Feb 23;118(6):237-8.

Lanas A, Panes J, Pique JM. Clinical implications of COX-1 and/or COX-2 inhibition for the distal gastrointestinal tract. Curr Pharm Des. 2003;9(27):2253-66.

Lanza FL. A guideline for the treatment and prevention of NSAID induced ulcers. Am J Gastroenterol 1998; 93:2037–2046.

Mantry P, Shah A, Sundaram U. Celecoxib associated esophagitis: review of gastrointestinal side effects from cox-2 inhibitors. J Clin Gastroenterol. 2003 Jul;37(1):61-3.

Muir H, et al. Effects of tiaprofenic acid and other NSAIDs on proteoglycan metabolism in articular cartilage explants. Drugs. 1988;35 Suppl 1:15-23.

Penglis PS. Differential regulation of prostaglandin E2 and thromboxane A2 production in human monocytes: implications for the use of cyclooxygenase inhibitors. J Immunol. 2000 Aug 1;165(3):1605-11.

Shield MJ. Anti-inflammatory drugs and their effects on cartilage synthesis and renal function. Eur J Rheumatol Inflamm. 1993;13(1):7-16.

Chapter 3
The Dreaded Rubber Glove

American Cancer Society website. www.cancer.org

Barnard RJ, Aronson WJ. Preclinical models relevant to diet, exercise, and cancer risk. Recent Results Cancer Res. 2005;166:47-61.

Colgan M. Protect Your Prostate. Apple Publishing Co. Ltd. Canada. 2000

Ekman P, et al. Estrogen receptors in human prostate: evidence for multiple binding sites. J Clin Endocrinol Metab.1983 Jul;57(1):166-76.

Freedland SJ, Aronson WJ. Examining the relationship between obesity and prostate cancer. Rev Urol. 2004 Spring;6(2):73-81.

Friedman AE. The Estradiol-Dihydrotestosterone model of prostate cancer. Theor Biol Med Model. 2005 Mar 18;2:10.

Gann PH, et al. A prospective evaluation of plasma prostate-specific antigen for detection of prostatic cancer. JAMA. 1995 Jan 25;273(4):289-94.

Hellerstedt BA, Pienta KJ (2002). The current state of hormonal therapy for prostate cancer. CA—A Cancer Journal for Clinicians, 52: 154–179.

Hoffman MA, et al. Is low serum free testosterone a marker for high grade prostate cancer? Journal of Urology. 2000 Mar;163(3):824-7.

Jian L, et al. Moderate physical activity and prostate cancer risk: a case-control study in China. Eur J Epidemiol. 2005;20(2):155-60.

Kaur Jaswinder. The number one `killer' cancer among men. New Straits Times. Sept.2, 2007.

Keetch DW, et al. Serial prostatic biopsies in men with persistently elevate serum prostate specific antigen values. The Journal of Urology 1994; 151(6):1571–1574.

Kreig M, Nass R, Tunn S. Effect of aging on endogenous level of 5 alpha-dihydrotestosterone, testosterone, estradiol, and estrone in epithelium and stroma of normal and hyperplastic human prostate. J Clin Endocrinol Metab. 1993 Aug;77(2):375-81.

Marks LS, et al. Effect of testosterone replacement therapy on prostate tissue in men with late-onset hypogonadism: a randomized controlled trial. JAMA. 2006 Nov 15;296(19):2351-61.

Morgentaler A, et al. Occult prostate cancer in men with low serum testosterone levels. Journal of the American Medical Association. 1996 Dec 18;276(23):1904-6.

Pechersky AV, et al. Androgen administration in middle-aged and ageing men: effects of oral testosterone undecanoate on dihydrotestosterone, oestradiol and prostate volume. Int J Androl. 2002 Apr;25(2):119-25.

Philips P. Reports at European Urology Congress reflect issues of interest to aging men. JAMA. 1998 May 6;279(17):1333-5.

Riedner CE, et al. Central obesity is an independent predictor of erectile dysfunction in older men. J Urol. 2006 Oct;176(4 Pt 1):1519-23.

Shibata Y, et al. Changes in the endocrine environment of the human prostate transition zone with aging: simultaneous quantitative analysis of prostatic sex steroids and comparison with human prostatic histological composition. Prostate. 2000 Jan;42(1):45-55.

Slater S, Oliver RT. Testosterone: its role in development of prostate cancer and potential risk from use as hormone replacement therapy. Drugs & Aging. 2000 Dec;17(6):431-9.

www.urologychannel.com: Testosterone Deficiency

Chapter 4
Addicted to Love

De Pergola G. The adipose tissue metabolism: role of testosterone and dehydroepiandrosterone. Int J Obes Relat Metab Disord. 2000 Jun;24 Suppl 2:S59-63.

Baba K, et al., Delayed testosterone replacement restores nitric oxide synthase-containing nerve fibres and the erectile response in rat penis. BJU Int. 2000 May;85(7):953-8.

Bhasin S., et al. Testosterone therapy in adult men with androgen deficiency syndromes: an endocrine society clinical practice guideline. J Clin Endocrinol Metab. 2006 Jun;91(6):1995-2010.

Billups KL, et al. Erectile Dysfunction Is a Marker for Cardiovascular Disease: Results of the Minority Health Institute Expert Advisory Panel. The Journal of Sexual Medicine. Volume 2 Issue 1 Page 40 - January 2005

El-Sakka AI, Hassoba HM. Age related testosterone depletion in patients with erectile dysfunction. J Urol. 2006 Dec;176(6 Pt 1):2589-93.

Gore J, Rajfer J. The role of serum testosterone testing: routine hormone analysis is an essential part of the initial screening of men with erectile dysfunction. Rev Urol. 2004 Fall;6(4):207-10.

Hwang Ti-S , et al. Combined use of androgen and sildenafil for hypogonadal patients unresponsive to sildenafil alone. International Journal of Impotence Research (2006) 18, 400–404.

Parker-Pope T. Viagra Is Misunderstood Despite Name Recognition. The Wall Street Journal online. Nov, 11, 2002.

Philips P. Reports at European Urology Congress reflect issues of interest to aging men. JAMA. 1998 May 6;279(17):1333-5.

Riedner CE, et al. Central obesity is an independent predictor of erectile dysfunction in older men. J Urol. 2006 Oct;176(4 Pt 1):1519-23.

Travison TG, et al. The relationship between libido and testosterone levels in aging men. J Clin Endocrinol Metab. 2006 Jul;91(7):2509-13. Epub 2006 May 2.

Yassin AA, et al. Testosterone undecanoate restores erectile function in a subset of patients with venous leakage: a series of case reports. J Sex Med. 2006 Jul;3(4):727-35.

Zhang XH, et al. Testosterone restores diabetes-induced erectile dysfunction and sildenafil responsiveness in two distinct animal models of chemical diabetes. J Sex Med. 2006 Mar;3(2):253-266

Zvara P, et al. Nitric oxide mediated erectile activity is a testosterone dependent event: a rat erection model. Int J Impot Res. 1995 Dec;7(4):209-19.

Chapter 5
Looking For Hair in All the Wrong Places

Able A. Why do some men lose their hair? Ezine Articles. Nov, 01, 2007.

Bang HJ, et al. Comparative studies on level of androgens in hair and plasma with premature male-pattern baldness. J Dermatol Sci. 2004 Feb;34(1):11-6.

Birch MP, Messenger AG. Genetic factors predispose to balding and non-balding in men. Eur J Dermatol. 2001 Jul;11(4):309-14.

Burke KE. Hair loss. What causes it and what can be done about it. Postgrad Med. 1989 May 1;85(6):52-73, 77.

Colin C. Men and Hair Loss: What Are Our Options? WebMD feature article.

Drake L, Hordinsky M et al. The effects of finasteride on scalp skin and serum androgen levels in men with androgenetic alopecia. J Am Acad Dermatol. 1999 Oct;41(4):550-4.

Ellis JA, Sinclair RD. Male pattern baldness: current treatments, future prospects. Drug Discov Today. 2008 Jul 7.

Ellis JA, et al. Baldness and the androgen receptor: the AR polyglycine repeat polymorphism does not confer susceptibility to androgenetic alopecia. Hum Genet. 2007 May;121(3-4):451-7.

Gautam M. Alopecia due to psychotropic medications. Ann Pharmacother. 1999 May;33(5):631-7.

Hadshiew IM, et al. Burden of hair loss: stress and the underestimated psychosocial impact of telogen effluvium and androgenetic alopecia. J Invest Dermatol. 2004 Sep;123(3):455-7.

Prager N, et al. A randomized, double-blind, placebo-controlled trial to determine the effectiveness of botanically derived inhibitors of 5-alpha-reductase in the treatment of androgenetic alopecia. J Altern Complement Med. 2002 Apr;8(2):143-52.

Price VH. Androgenetic alopecia in adolescents. Cutis. 2003 Feb;71(2):115-21.

Ryu HK, et al. Evaluation of androgens in the scalp hair and plasma of patients with male-pattern baldness before and after finasteride administration. Br J Dermatol. 2006 Apr;154(4):730-4.

Stene JJ. [Alopecia areata and treatment]. Rev Med Brux. 2004 Sep;25(4):A282-A285.

Chapter 6
Dude Look like a Lady

Abaci A, Buyukgebiz A. Gynecomastia: review. Pediatr Endocrinol Rev. 2007 Sep;5(1):489-99.

Bermant M. Causes of Gynecomastia. (Male Breast Enlargement, Gyno) - ww.plasticsurgery4u.com

Braunstein GD. Environmental gynecomastia. Endocr Pract. 2008 May-Jun;14(4):409-11.

Cakin N, Kamat D. Gynecomastia: evaluation and treatment recommendations for primary care providers. Clin Pediatr (Phila). 2007 Jul;46(6):487-90.

Comhaire F, Mahmoud A. Preventing diseases of the prostate in the elderly using hormones and nutriceuticals. Aging Male. 2004 Jun;7(2):155-69.

Lee SC, Ellis RJ. Male breast cancer during finasteride therapy. J Natl Cancer Inst 96(4):338 (2004).

Plourde PV, et al. Safety and efficacy of anastrozole for the treatment of pubertal gynecomastia: a randomized, double-blind, placebo-controlled trial. J Clin Endocrinol Metab. 2004 Sep;89(9):4428-33.

Pwlowski EJ, Nield LS. Gynecomastia and hypogonadism. Clin Pediatr (Phila). 2008 Apr;47(3):313-5

Sodi R, et al. Testosterone replacement-induced hyperprolactinaemia: case report and review of the literature. Ann Clin Biochem. 2005 Mar;42(Pt 2):153-9.

Sun ZY, Yin GQ. It is reasonable to do endocrine investigation in gynecomastia. Ann Plast Surg. 2008 Feb;60(2):228.

Gynecomastia: When Breasts Form in Males. Www.familydoctor.org

Hoffman J. What Are The Causes Of Gynecomastia? Ezine Articles. Aug, 29, 2007

www.wikipedia.com – gynecomastia

Chapter 7
Grumpy Old Men

Anderson P. Low Testosterone Levels Linked With Higher Risk for Depression. Medscape medical News. March 10, 2008

Almeida OP, et al. Low free testosterone concentration as a potentially treatable cause of depressive symptoms in older men. Arch Gen Psychiatry. 2008 Mar;65(3):283-9.

Amiaz R, Seidman SN. Testosterone and depression in men. Curr Opin Endocrinol Diabetes Obes. 2008 Jun;15(3):278-83.

Barrett-Connor E, et al. Bioavailable testosterone and depressed mood in older men: the Rancho Bernardo Study. J Clin Endocrinol Metab 1999; 84:573-77.

Conniff R. Testosterone under Attack. Web MD [feature from "Men's Health" Magazine] July 11, 2008.

Ebinger M, et al. Is there a neuroendocrinological rationale for testosterone as a therapeutic option in depression? J Psychopharmacol. 2008 Jun 18.

King BJ, Schmidt MA. Bio-Age: 10 Steps to a Younger You. CDG Books Canada. 2001.

Kratzik CW, et al. Mood changes, body mass index and bioavailable testosterone in healthy men: results of the Androx Vienna Municipality Study. BJU Int. 2007 Sep;100(3):614-8.

Margolese HC. The male menopause and mood: testosterone decline and depression in the aging male--is there a link? J Geriatr Psychiatry Neurol. 2000 Summer;13(2):93-101.

McIntyre RS, et al. Calculated bioavailable testosterone levels and depression in middle-aged men. Psychoneuroendocrinology. 2006 Oct;31(9):1029-35.

Orengo CA, et al. Male depression: a review of gender concerns and testosterone therapy. Geriatrics. 2004 Oct;59(10):24-30.

Pope HG et al. Testosterone gel supplementation for men with refractory depression: a randomized, placebo-controlled trial. Am J Psychiatry. 2003 Jan;160(1):105-11.

Regelson W, Colman C. The Superhormone Promise. Simon and Schuster, 1996; pages 132-135).

Seidman SN, Rabkin JG. Testosterone replacement therapy for hypogonadal men with SSRI-refractory depression. J Affect Disord. 1998 Mar;48(2-3):157-61.

Seidman SN. Testosterone deficiency and mood in aging men: pathogenic and therapeutic interactions. World J Biol Psychiatry. 2003 Jan;4(1):14-20.

Schutter DJ, et al   Administration of testosterone increases functional connectivity in a cortico-cortical depression circuit. J Neuropsychiatry Clin Neurosci. 2005 Summer;17(3):372-7.

Travison TG, et al. A population-level decline in serum testosterone levels in American men. J Clin Endocrinol Metab. 2007 Jan;92(1):196-202. Epub 2006 Oct 24.

Warner J. Low Testosterone Tied to Poor Health. Web MD Health News. July 5, 2006

Chapter 8
The Heart of the Matter

Akishita M, et al. Low testosterone level is an independent determinant of endothelial dysfunction in men. Hypertens Res. 2007 Nov;30(11):1029-34.

Attia N, et al. Increased phospholipids transfer protein activity associated with the impaired cellular cholesterol efflux in type 2 diabetic subjects with coronary disease. Tohoku J Exp. Med. 2007 Oct: 213(2): 129-37

Baker SK, Tarnopolsky MA. Statin myopathies: pathophysiologic and clinical perspectives. Clin Invest Med. 2001 Oct;24(5):258-72.

Bellosta S, et al. Safety of statins: focus on clinical pharmacokinetics and drug interactions. Circulation. 2004 Jun 15;109(23 Suppl 1):11150-7.

Brunzell JD, et al. Lipoprotein management in patients with cardiometabolic risk: consensus statement from the American Diabetes Association and the American College of Cardiology Foundation. Diabetes Care April, 2008. 31: 811-822

Dobrzycki S, et al. An assessment of correlations between endogenous sex hormone levels and the extensiveness of coronary heart disease and the ejection fraction of the left ventricle in males. J Med Invest. 2003 Aug;50(3-4):162-9.

Fogari R, et al. Plasma testosterone in isolated systolic hypertension Hypertension. 2003 Oct;42(4). Epub 2003 Sep 15.

Galbraith D, et al. Biology, McGraw-Hill Ryerson, Toronto, Ontario, 2003, p. 314

Gould DC, et al. Hypoandrogen-metabolic syndrome: a potentially common and underdiagnosed condition in men. Int J Clin Pract. 2007 Feb:61(2):341-4

Gorman C, Park A. "The Fires Within," www.TIME.com, posted Feb. 15, 2004

Hak AE, et al. Low levels of endogenous androgens increase the risk atherosclerosis in elderly men: The Rotterdam Study. J Clin Endocrinol Metab. 2002 Aug;87(8):3632-9

Jones RD, et al. Testosterone and atherosclerosis in aging men: purported association and clinical implications. Am J Cardiovasc Drugs. 2005;5(3):141-54.

Kang SM, et al. Effect of oral administration of testosterone on brachial arterial vasoreactivity in men with coronary artery disease. Am J Cardiol. 2002 Apr 1;89(7):862-4.

Kannel WB, et al. Is the relation of systolic blood pressure to risk of cardiovascular disease continuous and graded, or are there critical values? Hypertension, 2003 Oct:42(4):453-6. Epub 2003 Sep 15

Mader SS. Inquiry into life, Tenth Edition, McGraw Hill Higher Education, New York, NY, 2003, p. 242

Malkin CJ, et al. Testosterone replacement in hypogonadal men with angina improves ischaemic threshold and quality of life. Heart. 2004 Aug;90(8):871-6.

Park A. "Beyond Cholesterol," TIME Canada, November 25, 2002, p. 40

Pasternak RC, et al. ACC/AHA/NHLBI clinical advisory on the use and safety of statins. Circulation. 2002 Aug 20;106(8):1024-8.

Pugh PJ, et al. Testosterone: a natural tonic for the failing heart? J Med 2000; 93: 689-694

Ridker P. Centre for Science in the Public Interest, "New Clue to an Old Killer, Nutrition Action Health Letter; Canadian edition, Vol. 27, No. 7, Sept. 2000, p. 3

Stryer, L. Biochemistry, 4th Ed. (in English), New York: W.H. Freeman & Co., 1995. 280, 703

Svartberg J. Epidemiology: testosterone and the metabolic syndrome. Int J Impot Res. 2007 Mar-Apr;19(2):124-8.

Turhan S, et al. The association between androgen levels and premature coronary artery disease in men. Coron Artery Dis. 2007 May: 18(3):159-62

Chapter 9
Stress and Immunity

Arai MH, et al. "The effects of long-term endurance training on the immune and endocrine systems of elderly men: the role of cytokines and anabolic hormones. Immunity & Ageing 2006, 3:9

Butcher SK, et al. Raised cortisol:DHEAS ratios in the elderly after injury: potential impact upon neutrophil function and immunity. Aging Cell. 2005 Dec;4(6):319-24.

Borghese, C.M., et al. "Cortisol, the Muscle Eater." Brain Res Bull 31 (1993):697–700.

Cruess DG, et al. Cognitive-behavioral stress management buffers decreases in dehydroepiandrosterone sulfate (DHEA-S) and increases in the cortisol/DHEA-S ratio and reduces mood disturbance and perceived stress among HIV-seropositive men. Psychoneuroendocrinology. 1999 Jul;24(5):537-49.

Elmlinger MW, et al. Endocrine alterations in the aging male. Clin Chem Lab Med. 2003 Jul;41(7):934-41.

Ferrari E, et al. Age-Related changes of the hypothalamic-pituitary-adrenal axis: pathophysiological correlates. Euo J Endocrin. 2001 Apr;144(4):319- 29.

Hansen PA, et al. DHEA protects against visceral obesity and muscle insulin resistance in rats fed a high-fat diet. Am J Physiol. 1997 Nov;273(5 Pt 2):R1704-8.

Jefferies WM. Cortisol and immunity. Med Hypotheses. 1991 Mar;34(3):198-208.

Lane JD. Neuroendocrine responses to caffeine in the work environment. Psychosom Med. 1994 May-Jun;56(3):267-70.

Lane JD, et al. Caffeine affects cardiovascular and neuroendocrine activation at work and home. Psychosom Med. 2002 Jul-Aug;64(4):595-603.

Lardy, H, Partridge, B, Kneer N, and Wei, Y. Ergosteroids: Induction of thermogenic enzymes in liver of rats treated with steroids derived from dehydroepiandrosterone. Proc. Natl. Acad. Sci. USA, 1995; 92: 6617-6619.

Jedrzejuk D, et al. Dehydroepiandrosterone replacement in healthy men with age-related decline of DHEA-S: effects on fat distribution, insulin sensitivity and lipid metabolism. Aging Male. 2003 Sep;6(3):151-6.

Lovallo, W.R., et al. Stress-like adrenocorticotropin responses to caffeine in young healthy men. Pharmacology, Biochemistry and Behavior. 1996 Nov;55(3):365-9.

Morgan CA, et al. Relationships among plasma dehydroepiandrosterone sulfate and cortisol levels, symptoms of dissociation, and objective performance in humans exposed to acute stress. Arch Gen Psychiatry. 2004 Aug;61(8):819-25.

Pelletier, Kenneth. Mind as Healer, Mind as Slayer. Stanford University Press, 2002.

Testosterone, Stress May Not Suppress Immune System After All, Science Daily. Oct, 7, 1999.

Wilmore J, Costill D. Physiology of Sport and Exercise. Champaign, IL: Human Kinetics; 1999.

Part 2
The Education and Reinvention of Fred

Chapter 10
We Really Are What – And How - We Eat

King, B., Fat Wars Action Planner, Wiley Canada, Toronto, 2003.

Cassidy, C.M. "Nutrition and Health in Agriculturists and Hunter-Gatherers: A Case Study of Two Prehistoric Populations." Nutritional Anthropology, Pleasantville, New York: 117-145.

Challem, J., et al. Syndrome X: The Complete Nutritional Program to Prevent and
Reverse Insulin Resistance. New York: John Wiley & Sons, 2001.

Eaton, S.B, et al. "An Evolutionary Perspective Enhances Understanding of Human Nutritional Requirements." Journal of Nutrition 126 (1996): 1732-1740.

Hanis T, et al. Effects of dietary trans-fatty acids on reproductive performance of Wistar rats. Br J Nutr. 1989 May;61(3):519-29.

Hellström, L. Studies on catecholamine function in human fat cells, Föreläsningssalen, Medicingatan. Dec., 6 1996.

Hill PB, Wynder EL. Effect of a vegetarian diet and dexamethasonenon plasma prolactin, testosterone and dehydroepiandrosterone in men and women. Cancer Lett 1979 Sep;7(5):273-82.

Holm C. Molecular mechanisms regulating hormone-sensitive lipase and lipolysis. Biochem Soc Trans. 2003 Dec;31(Pt 6):1120-4.

Key TJ, et al. Testosterone, sex hormone-binding globulin, calculated free testosterone, and oestradiol in male vegans and omnivores. Br J Nutr. 1990 Jul;64(1):111-9.

King, B.J. Fat Wars: 45 days to Transform Your Body. Toronto: Macmillan, 2002.

Longcope, C., et al. "Diet and Sex Hormone-Binding Globulin," J Clin Endocrinol Metab, 2000, 85: 1, 293-6.

Mutungi BG, et al. Dietary cholesterol from eggs increases plasma HDL cholesterol in overweight men consuming a carbohydrate-restricted diet. J Nutr, 2008 Feb;138(2):272-6.

Pauling L, How to Live Longer and Feel Better, Avon books, Inc., New York, NY, 1986, p. 49.

Riechman SE, et al. Statins and dietary and serum cholesterol are associated with increased lean mass following resistance training. J Gerontol A Biol Sci Med Sci, 2007 Oct;62(10):1164-71

Shahbazpour N, et al. Early alterations in serum creatine kinase and total cholesterol following high intensity eccentric muscle actions. J Sports Med Phys Fitness, 2004;44:193-199.

Sallinen J, et al. Dietary intake, serum hormones, muscle mass and strength during strength training in 49-73 year-old-men. Int J Sports Med, 2007 Dec;28(12) 1070-6.

Taskinen, M.R., and E. Nikkila. "Lipoprotein Lipase of Adipose Tissue and Skeletal Muscle in Human Obesity" Metabolism 30 (1981): 810-817.

Wang C, et al. Low-Fat, High-Fiber Diet Decreased Serum and Urine Androgens in Men. J Clin Endocrinol Metab, 2005 Jun;90(6):3550-9.

Zock PL, Mensink RP. Dietary trans-fatty acids and serum lipoproteins in humans. Curr Opin Lipidol. 1996 Feb;7(1):34-7.

www.wikipedia.org/wiki/Trans_fat

Chapter 11
Blood, Sweat and Testosterone: The Secret to Efficient and Effective Exercise

Alessio, H.M.; Exercise-induced Oxidative Stress, Med Sci Sports Exerc, (Feb 1993), 25:2, 218–24.

Aniansson A., et al; Effect of a Training Program for Pensioners on Condition and Muscular Strength, Arch Gerontol Geriatr, 3 (Oct 1984):229–41.

Batmanghelidj, F.; Your Body's Many Cries for Water, Falls Church, VA: Global Health Solutions, 1998.

Bhasin, S., et al. "The Effects of Supraphysiologic Doses of Testosterone on Muscle Size and Strength in Normal Men," New Engl J Med, July 1996, 335, no. 1: 1-7.

Blomstrand E, Saltin B. BCAA intake affects protein metabolism in muscle after but not during exercise in humans. Am J Physiol Endocrinol Metab. 2001 Aug;281(2):E365-74.

Borst S.E., et al; "Growth Hormone, Exercise, and Aging: The Future of Therapy for the Frail Elderly," J Am Geriatr Soc,, 42:5 (May, 1998):528–35.

Brsheim, E., et al; "Adrenergic Control of Post-exercise Metabolism," Acta Physiol Scand, 162 (Mar 1998):313–23.

Burke, ER.; Optimal Muscle Recovery, Avery Publishing Group, 1999.

Carlson, LA., et al; "Studies on Blood Lipids During Exercise," J Lab Clin Med, 61 (1963):724–729.

Coggan A.R. et al. "Fat Metabolism During High-Intensity Exercise in Endurance-Trained and Untrained Men," Metabolism 49 (2000):122–8.

Colgan, M; The New Nutrition, Vancouver: Apple Publishing, 1995.

Fernández Pastor V.J., et al; "Function of Growth Hormone in the Human Energy Continuum During Physical Exertion," Rev Esp Fisiol, 47 (Dec 1991):223–9.

Gotshalk, LA, et.al. Pituitary-gonadal hormonal responses of multi-set vs. single -set resistance exercise. Journal of Strength and Conditioning Research.

10(4):286. 1996

Hagberg J.M., et al; "Metabolic Responses to Exercise in Young and Older Athletes and Sedentary Men", J Appl Physiol, 65 (Aug 1988):900–8.

Karlsson J.; Metabolic Adaptations to Exercise: A Review of Potential Beta-adrenoceptor Antagonist Effects, Am J Cardiol, 55 (Apr 1985):48D–58D.

Kennedy R. The Natural Anabolic Steroid (or TNAS); The Doctor's Medical Library.

Kostka T. "Aging, Physical Activity and Free Radicals" Pol Merkuriusz Lek, 7 (Oct 1999):202–4.

Woods J.A., et al; "Effects of 6 Months on Moderate Aerobic Exercise Training on Immune Function in the Elderly," Mech Ageing Dev, 109 (June 1999):1–19

Chapter 12
Ultimate Male Solutions: The Top Nutrients for Male Health

Whey Protein Isolate

Baruchel S., Vaiu G., In vitro selective modulation of cellular glutathione by a humanized native milk protein isolate in normal cells and rat mammary carcinoma model. Anticancer Res. 1996 May-Jun;16(3A):1095-9.

Bounous G., Gold P., The biological activity of undenatured dietary whey proteins: role of glutathione. Clin Invest Med. 1991 Aug;14(4):296-309.

Bounous G., The immunoenhancing property of dietary whey protein concentrate. Clin Invest Med. 1988 Aug;11(4):271-8

Bounous G, et al. The influence of dietary whey protein on tissue glutathione and the diseases of aging In: Clin Invest Med (1989 Dec) 12(6):343-9

Dangin et al, The rate of protein digestion affects protein gain differently during aging in humans. J Physiol, June, 2003, 549(2):17(1):27-33

Kennedy R.S., et al. The use of a whey protein concentrate in the treatment of patients with metastatic carcinoma: a phase I-II clinical study. Anticancer Res. 1995 Nov-Dec;15(6B):2643-9.

Lands LC, Grey VL and Smountas AA. Effect of a cysteine donor on muscular performance. J Appl Physiol. 1999 Oct;87(4):1381-5.

McIntosh G.H., et al. Dairy proteins protect against dimethylhydrazine-induced intestinal cancers in rats. J Nutr. 1995 Apr;125(4):809-16.

Takada Y, et al. Whey protein stimulated the proliferation and differentiation of osteoblastic MC3T3-E1 cells. Biochem Biophys Res Commun. 1996 Jun

14;223(2):445-9.

Travison, TG, et al. A population-level decline in serum testosterone levels in American men. J. Clin Endocrin Metab 92:196-202.

www.womenshealth.gov Aging Male Syndrome

Maca

Cicero AF. Hexanic Maca extract improves rat sexual performance more effectively than methanolic and chloroformic Maca extracts. Andrologia. 2002 Jun;34(3):177-9.

Gasco M , et al. Dose-response effect of red maca (Lepidium meyenii) on benign prostatic hyperplasia induced by testosterone enanthate . Phytomedicine . 2007;14(7-8):460-464.

Muhammad I, et al. Constituents of Lepidium meyenii 'maca'. Phytochemistry. 2002 Jan;59(1):105-10.

Gonzales GF, et al. Effect of Lepidium meyenii (MACA) on sexual desire and its absent relationship with serum testosterone levels in adult healthy men. Andrologia, 2002 Dec;34(6):367-72.

Gonzales GF, et al. Lepidium meyenii (maca) improved semen parameters in adult men . Asian J Androl . 2001;3(4):301-303.

Gonzales GF, et al. Red maca (Lepidium meyenii) reduced prostate size in rats . Reprod Biol Endocrinol . 2005;3:5.

Oshima M , et al. Effects of Lepidium meyenii Walp and Jatropha macrantha on blood levels of estradiol-17 beta, progesterone, testosterone and the rate of embryo implantation in mice . J Vet Med Sci . 2003;65(10):1145-1146.

Valentova K, et al. Prospective Andean Crops for the Prevention of Chronic Diseases. Biomed Papers 2003. 147(2), 119-130.

Zhang Y, et al. Effect of ethanol extract of Lepidium meyenii Walp. on osteoporosis in ovariectomized rat . J Ethnopharmacol . 2006;105(1-2):274-279.

Zheng BL , et al. Effect of a lipidic extract from Lepidium meyenii on sexual behavior in mice and rats . Urology. 2000;55(4):598-602.

Tongkat Ali

Ang, HH: Eurycoma longifolia Jack enhances libido in sexually experienced male rats Exp Anim 1997 Oct;46(4):287-90

Ang HH, Cheang HS. Effects of Eurycoma longifolia jack on laevator ani muscle in both uncastrated and testosterone-stimulated castrated intact male rats. Arch Pharm Res. 2001 Oct;24(5):437-40.

Ang HH, Lee KL, Kioshi M. Eurycoma longifolia Jack enhances sexual motivation in middle-aged male mice. J Basic Clin Physiol Pharmacol. 2003;14(3):301-8

Cheang HS et al., Effects of Eurycoma longifolia Jack (Tongkat ali) on the initiation of sexual performance of inexperienced castrated male rats. Exp Anim 2000 Jan;49(1):35-8

Hamzah S, Yusof A. The Ergogenic Effects Of Eurycoma Longifolia Jack: A Pilot Study Br J Sports Med 2003;37:464-470

Ismail MTM. Proceedings paper: Asian Congress of Sexology. 2002.

Kilham, C. Tongkat Ali The Youth-promoting Herb, Total Health; Jun/Jul2004, Vol. 26 Issue 3, p52-53

Ngai TH et al. Aphrodisiac evaluation in non-copulator male rats after chronic administration of Eurycoma longifolia. Fundam Clin Pharmacol 2001 Aug;15(4):265-8

Chrysin

Brown GA, et al. Effects of anabolic precursors on serum testosterone concentrations and adaptations to resistance training in young men. Int J Sport Nutr Exerc Metab 2000;10:340-59.

Campbell DR, Kurzer MS. Flavonoid inhibition of aromatase enzyme activity in human preadipocytes.
J Steroid Biochem Mol Biol. 1993 Sep;46(3):381-8.

Izquierdo M, et al. Effects of strength training on muscle power and serum hormones in middle-aged and older men. J App Physiol. 2001 Apr;90(4): 1497-507.

Jeong HJ, et al. Inhibition of aromatase activity by flavonoids. Arch Pharm Res. 1999; 22:309-312

Vogel P. Improve Your Sex Life and Protect Against Heart Attack. Life Extension Magazine, May 2003.

www.labtestsonline.com: Sex Hormone Binding Globulin

Beta Sitosterol

Awad AB, et al. In vitro and in vivo (SCID mice) effects of phytosterols on the growth and dissemination of human prostate cancer PC-3 cells. Eur J Cancer

Prev. 2001 Dec;10(6):507-13.

Berges RR, et al. Randomised, placebo-controlled, double-blind clinical trial of beta-sitosterol in patients with benign prostatic hyperplasia. Beta-sitosterol Study Group. Lancet, 1995 Jun 17;345(8964):1529-32

Braeckman J. The extract of Serenoa repens in the treatment of benign prostatic hyperplasia: A multicenter open study Current Therapeutic Research, vol 55 (1994).

Duan RD. Anticancer compounds and sphingolipid metabolism in the colon. In Vivo. 2005 Jan-Feb;19(1):293-300

Katz AE. Dr. Katz's Guide to Prostate Health, From Conventional to Holistic Therapies. Freedom Press, 2006.

Sarkar FH, et al. Bax translocation to mitochondria is an important event in inducing apoptotic cell death by indole-3-carbinol (I3C) treatment of breast cancer cells. J Nutr 2003 Jul;133(7 Suppl):2434S-2439S.

von Holtz RL, et al. Beta-Sitosterol activates the sphingomyelin cycle and induces apoptosis in LNCaP human prostate cancer cells. Nutr Cancer. 1998;32(1):8-12.

Wright J, Lenard L. Maximize Your Vitality and Potency For Men Over 40. Smart Publications, Petaluma CA, 1999. Chapter 3.

Indoles

Bradlow, HL, et al. Phytochemicals as modulators of cancer risk. Advances in Experimental Medicine and Biology, 1999, 472, 207-221

Bradlow, HL, et al. Multifunctional aspects of the action of indole-3-carbinol as an antitumor agent. Annals of the New York Academy of Sciences, 1999, 889, 204-21

Cohen, JH, et al. Fruit and vegetable intakes and prostate cancer risk. Journal of the National Cancer Institute, 2000, 92, 61-68

Farnsworth WE. Estrogen in the etiopathogenesis of BPH. Prostate, 1999, 41:263-74.

Hecht SS, et al. Effects of cruciferous vegetable consumption on urinary metabolites of the tobacco-specific lung carcinogen 4-(methylnitrosamino)-1-(3- pyridyl)-1-butanone in Singapore Chinese. Cancer Epidemiol Bio Prev. 2004 JuN;13(6):997-04.

Hsu JC, et al. Indole-3-carbinol inhibition of androgen receptor expression and downregulation of androgen responsiveness in human prostate cancer cells. 2005 Nov;26(11):1896-904.

McAlindon TE, et al. Indole-3-carbinol in women with SLE: effect on estrogen metabolism and disease activity. Lupus. 2001;10(11):779-83.

Sarkar FH, et al. Bax translocation to mitochondria is an important event in inducing apoptotic cell death by indole-3-carbinol (I3C) treatment of breast cancer cells. J Nutr 2003 Jul;133(7 Suppl):2434S-2439S.

Sarkar FH, et al. Indole-3-carbinol and prostate cancer. J Nutr. 2004 Dec;134(12 Suppl):3493S-3498S

Zhang J, et al. Indole-3-carbinol induces a G1 cell cycle arrest and inhibits prostate-specific antigen production in human LNCaP prostate carcinoma cells. 2003 Dec 1;98(11):2511-20

Stinging Nettle Root

Hyrb D et al. The effect of extracts of the roots of the stinging nettle (Urtica dioca) on the interaction of SHBG with its receptor on human prostatic membranes. Planta Med, 1995, 61:31-32.

Jellin J. Natural Medicines Comprehensive DataBase, Pharmacist's Letter

Katz AE. Dr. Katz's Guide to Prostate Health, From Conventional to Holistic Therapies. Freedom Press, 2006

Konrad L, et al. Antiproliferative effect on human prostate cancer cells by a stinging nettle root (Urtica dioica) extract. Planta Med 2000;66:44-7.

Mittman P. Randomized, double-blind study of freeze-dried Urtica dioica in the treatment of allergic rhinitis.Planta Med 1990;56:44-7

Randall C, et al. Nettle sting of Urtica dioica for joint pain--an exploratory study of this complementary therapy. Compl Ther Med 1999;7:126–31.

Schottner M et al. Lignans from the roots of Urtica dioca and their metabolites bind to human sex hormone binding globulin (SHBG). Planta Med 1997, 63:529-32. 9.

Vontobel H, et al. Results of a double-blind study on the effectiveness of ERU (extractum radicis urticae) capsules in conservative treatment of benign prostatic hyperplasia. Urologe 1985;24:49–51

Epimedium (Horny Goat Weed)

Bensky D, et al. Chinese Herbal Medicine Materia Medica. Revised Edition, Seattle: Eastland Press, 1992.

Chen JK, Chen TT. Chinese Medical Herbology and Pharmacology. City of

Industry, CA: Art of Medicine Press, Inc., 2004.

Liao HJ, et al. Effect of Epimedium sagittatum on quality of life and cellular immunity in patients of hemodialysis maintenance. Zhongguo Zhong Xi Yi Jie He Za Zhi 1995;15:202-4

Liu J, et al. Clinical Observation on 271 Cases of Non-Small Lung Cancer Treated with Yifei Kangliu Yin (Jin Fu Kang). Chinese Journal of Integrated Traditional and Western Medicine 2001; 7(4):247-250.

Mao H, et al. Experimental studies of icariin on anticancer mechanism. Zhong Yao Cai 2000; 23(9):554-556.

Yap SP, et al. New estrogenic prenylflavone from Epimedium brevicornum inhibits the growth of breast cancer cells. Planta Med 2005;71:114-9.

Lycopene

Giovannucci et. al. A prospective study of tomato products, lycopene, and prostate cancer risk. Journal of the National

Hadley et. al. Tomatoes, lycopene, and prostate cancer: Progress and promise. Experimental Biology and Medicine 227:869-880 (2002)

Katz AE. Dr. Katz's Guide to Prostate Health, From Conventional to Holistic Therapies. Freedom Press, 2006.

Sarkar FH, et al. Bax translocation to mitochondria is an important event in inducing apoptotic cell death by indole-3-carbinol (I3C) treatment of breast cancer cells. J Nutr 2003 Jul;133(7 Suppl):2434S-2439S.

Schwarz et al. Lycopene Inhibits Disease Progression in Patients with Benign Prostate Hyperplasia J. Nutr. 138:49-53, January 2008

Zinc

Ali H, et al. Relationship of serum and seminal plasma zinc levels and serum testosterone in oligospermic and azoospermic infertile men. J Coll Physicians Surg Pak. 2005 Nov;15(11):671-3.

Wei Sheng Yan Jiu. [The effects of zinc deficiency and testosterone supplement on testosterone synthesis and skeletal muscle of rats], 1997 May;26(3):211-5.

Kilic M. Effect of fatiguing bicycle exercise on thyroid hormone and testosterone levels in sedentary males supplemented with oral zinc. Neuro Endocrinol Lett. 2007 Oct;28(5):681-5.

Kvist U et. al. Sperm nuclear zinc, chromatin stability, and male fertility. Scanning Microsc. 1987 Sep;1(3):1241-7

Prasad AS et. al. Zinc status and serum testosterone levels of healthy adults. Nutrition, Volume 12, No.5, 1996, pp. 344-348.

Sarkar FH, et al. Bax translocation to mitochondria is an important event in inducing apoptotic cell death by indole-3-carbinol (I3C) treatment of breast cancer cells. J Nutr 2003 Jul;133(7 Suppl):2434S-2439S.

Chapter 13
Testing, One, Two, Three

Katz AE. Dr. Katz's Guide to Prostate Health, From Conventional to Holistic Therapies. Freedom Press, 2006.

Travison TG, et al. A population-level decline in serum testosterone levels in American men. J Clin Endocrinol Metab. 2007 Jan;92(1):196-202.

Wright J, Lenard L. Maximize Your Vitality and Potency For Men Over 40. Smart Publications, Petaluma CA, 1999. Chapter 3.

Roberts E. Pregneolone—from Selye to Alzheimer and a model of the pregnenolone sulfate binding site on the GABAA receptor. Biochem Pharmacol. 1995 Jan 6;49(1):1-16.

Mayo W, et al. Individual differences in cognitive aging: implication of pregnenolone sulfate. Prog Neurobiol. 2003 Sep;71(1):43-8.

Lam P et. al. Empirical estimation of free testosterone from testosterone and sex hormone binding globulin immunoassays. European Journal of Endocrinology 2005 Vol. 152, Issue 3, 471-478.

Muti P, et al. Urinary estrogen metabolites and prostate cancer: a case-control study in the United States. Cancer Causes Control. 2002 Dec;13(10): 947-55.

www.womenshealth.gov/mens/sexual/ams.cfm
www.labtestsonline.org/understanding/analytes/testosterone/glance.html
www.womenshealth.gov/mens/sexual/ams.cfm
www.labtestsonline.org/understanding/analytes/lipid/glance.html
www.lef.org/magazine/mag2006/nov2006_report_hormone_01.htm
www.lef.org/magazine/mag2005/jun2005_report_hormone_01.htm
www.lef.org/magazine/mag2005/jun2005_report_hormone_02.htm
labtestsonline.org/understanding/analytes/psa/test.html
labtestsonline.org/understanding/analytes/crp/test.html
labtestsonline.org/understanding/analytes/dheas/test.html
www.labtestsonline.org/understanding/analytes/testosterone/glance.html

www.BeerBellyBlues.com